The Moral Challenges of Health Care Management

The Moral Challenges of Health Care Management

John R. Griffith

Health Administration Press
Ann Arbor, Michigan 1993

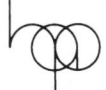

Copyright © 1993 by John R. Griffith. Printed in the United States of America. All rights reserved. This book or parts thereof may not be reproduced in any form without written permission of the publisher. Opinions and views expressed in this book are those of the author and do not necessarily reflect those of the Foundation of the American College of Healthcare Executives.

96 95 94 93 92   5 4 3 2 1

Library of Congress Cataloging-in-Publication Data

Griffith, John R.
  The moral challenges of health care management / John R. Griffith.
    p. cm.
  Includes bibliographical references.
  ISBN 0-910701-93-8 (hardbound : alk. paper)
  1. Health services administration—Moral and ethical aspects. 2. Health services administration—Moral and ethical aspects—Case studies. I. Title.
  [DNLM: 1. Delivery of Health Care—organization & administration. 2. Ethics, Medical. 3. Health facilities—organization & administration. W 50 G853m]
RA394.G75   1993   362.1′068—dc20
DNLM/DLC for Library of Congress   92-48699 CIP

The paper used in this publication meets the minimum requirements of American National Standard for Information Sciences—Permanence of Paper for Printed Library Materials, ANSI Z39.48-1984. ∞™

Health Administration Press
A division of the Foundation of the
  American College of Healthcare Executives
1021 East Huron Street
Ann Arbor, Michigan 48104-9990
(313) 764-1380

*To all those health care managers
who accepted the moral challenge:
There have been many, and our world
is better as a result of their effort.*

Contents

Foreword by David C. Thomasma xi

Preface xix

Acknowledgments xxii

Suggested Readings xxiii

Part I   Introduction

Ethical Commitments of Health Care Managers 3
    Humanity as an End 3
    About This Book 6
    Notes 9

Appendix I.A
American College of Healthcare Executives
    Code of Ethics 11
    Ethical Policy Statement: Impaired Healthcare Executives 16

Appendix I.B
American Hospital Association
    Ethical Conduct for Health Care Institutions 18

Part II Theories of Moral Obligation

Case 1
Abortion Policy at XYZ Community Hospital 25

Case 2
Baby Doe: Care of Severely Damaged Neonates 29

Part II Commentary
The Diversity of Theories of Moral Obligation and the
Implications for Health Care Management 39

    What Theories of Moral Obligation Are and How They Differ 40

        The nature of theories of moral obligation   *40*
        The types of theories of moral obligation   *41*
        Act versus rule applications   *42*
        The origins of theories of moral obligation   *42*

    Application of Theories of Moral Obligation 43

    Dealing with Conflict in Theories of Moral Obligation 46

        Consequences of unresolved conflict   *46*
        Some actions to avoid   *46*
        Options for the health care executive   *47*

Notes to Part II 50

Part III Conflicting *Prima Facie* Obligations

Case 3
Providing References 53

Case 4
The Doctor, the Patient, and the DRG 57

Case 5
Terminating the Employment Contract—The Abortion Case,
Part Two 61

Case 6
The End of Life: Assisting Families and Clinical Personnel with
Terminal Care 63

Case 7
Tough Transplant Questions Raised by Baby Jesse Case 67

Part III Commentary
Dealing with Conflicting Moral Obligations—Negotiating the
Slippery Slope 73

    How Conflicting Obligations Arise 73

    Relationship between *Prima Facie* Conflicts and Nonmoral
    Management 74

    How Good Nonmoral Management Contributes to
    Solving the Cases 75

        Reference letters (Case 3)   75
        DRG management (Case 4)   76
        The moral grounds for resignation and termination
            (Case 5)   77
        Terminal care (Case 6)   78
        Transplants (Case 7)   82

    A Theory for Dealing with *Prima Facie* Conflicts 83

        Required assumptions about moral obligations   83
        Guiding the organization's *prima facie* selections   84
        Applying the rules for managing conflicting obligations
            to clinical areas   88

    Notes 90

Part IV   Improving Virtue

Case 8
The Question of Venial Sins 93

Case 9
Dr. Burt of St. Elizabeth's 95

Case 10
Commodore Quinn and Captain Hodges 103

Case 11
John McCabe and Blue Cross and Blue Shield of Michigan 111

Part IV Commentary
Building the Virtuous Health Care Corporation 125

The Concept of Moral Virtue 125
Can Nonmoral Actions Promote Moral Virtue? A Review
of the Cases 126
Why Lead a Moral Life? The Personal Promotion of
Moral Virtue 130
When Is Command Moral? 132
    The moral justification for authority   *133*
    The moral obligation of authority   *134*
Is Punishment Wise? The Uses of Blame and Retribution in
Management 134
Can a Manager Be a Moral Leader? 135
    Promoting moral virtue by example   *136*
    Nonmoral actions that promote moral behavior   *136*

Part IV Epilogue

Follow-up on the Cases 141
  St. Elizabeth's 141
  Commodore Quinn and Captain Hodges 141
  Blue Cross and Blue Shield of Michigan 145
Notes to Part IV 149

About the Author 153

Foreword

John Griffith begins and ends this book with humility. This humility is important, as important as the many insights he brings to the newly shaped discipline of health care management ethics. It is important because of the horrendously complex pressures and interests that are brought to bear today on the task of managing and directing our health care institutions.

The challenges of managing a health care institution or system today are almost overwhelming. Consider the changes in the environment. Today almost every decision must be weighed against the competition. Competitiveness creates fissures in what was once a unified profession. Competitiveness also pushes institutional loyalty over an internal morality of the profession that would instead stress an individual's duties of moral leadership. The latter duty would transcend institutional loyalty. Such leadership would be exercised for oneself and for everyone in the field, regardless of institution.

A good example of the conflict institutional loyalty creates might be a plan, such as one proposed in Illinois in 1992, to tax hospitals whose burden for care of the poor is less (i.e., wealthier hospitals) and funnel that money to those hospitals that bear a proportionately greater burden of caring for the poor (i.e., urban hospitals in large cities). As the politics of such a plan are worked out, executives find themselves allied against one another. Those in the wealthier, suburban hospitals fight against the plan, while their brothers and sisters in the poorer hospitals struggle on behalf of the merits of the plan. Legislators find themselves in a quandary because of the divided and contentious message created by institutional loyalties.

Or think of increasingly complex personnel issues, where doing the right thing for one's employees also means checking with other institutions about their activities in this regard. Consider other issues like pleasing the board and carrying out its requirements for responsible leadership, ensuring that the staff of the hospital or nursing home or social service are not victims of ineptitude in managing resources and caring for patients, enabling employees to speak their consciences, and, very importantly, providing mechanisms for resolving disputes about the mission and philosophy of the institution.

These illustrations describe a major change and its major challenges. The American College of Healthcare Executives' Ethical Policy Statement on Responsibility to Employees, issued by the College in March 1992, describes the emerging health care environment as follows:

> The structure of modern health care organizations has undergone a dramatic change, one through which the organizations of health care delivery were fundamentally altered. In the past these organizations, and the responsibilities of those who managed them, were organized around providing a decent environment in which the caregivers could practice their craft virtually untended. Today, by contrast, the organizations themselves are held publically accountable in moral and legal terms for the quality and effectiveness of the care.
>
> Thus, a paradigm shift has occurred. In the past we were accustomed to thinking in terms of the individual doctor-patient relationship. Today, we must rethink the delivery of care as a community of caregivers, with third-party interests, working within a close-knit and mutually supportive environment. When any part of this dynamic fails, the quality of care and the moral stature of the institution collapses.

Given this complexity of duties and environments, let us look more carefully at some of the issues John Griffith raises.

First, is there an internal morality of the profession? He suggests that there is. It is based, in his view, on deontological duties individuals have toward other persons. Health care managers willingly take on these duties. Because of this commitment to those within the institution, they must take care to live an exemplary life, setting the standards of behavior to be followed in the institution. One might develop this duty even further by arguing that health care managers share not only in those features of business ethics that require honesty and integrity but also in the internal morality of health care itself. In this view, health care managers would take as their primary value the good of the patient and detail its implications in every aspect of institutional management.

Second, how does the manager care for the self? John Griffith suggests that the nurturing of the self is essential in developing one's ethics and one's posture within and on behalf of institutions. Only persons of ethical maturity should consider entering the profession. Ethical maturity might be defined as the ability to weather criticism and pressure in order to do what is right and good. Individuals considering any management position must have strongly delineated goals and clearly defined values as well as the ability to carry these out. These characteristics can create tremendous stress when values come into conflict. Leadership demands an ability to articulate how the values are in conflict and how the resolution properly respects a hierarchy of values.

Third, what are the requirements to care for the staff? The Code of Ethics of the American College of Healthcare Executives (ACHE) was recently revised to explicitly address the health care executive's duty to employees of the institution. First and foremost, the manager must develop an environment that is conducive to underscoring the ethical conduct and behavior of employees. Providing the proper example is only the first step in this process. The next must surely be ensuring that individuals may freely express their ethical concerns without jeopardizing their jobs. And the next step would be providing mechanisms for the discussion of such concerns and for addressing and redressing them, so employees know where to turn for support.

The manager would have to be vigilant to root out any coercive mechanisms that might make it convenient for employees of the health care institution to perform illegal or immoral acts. Particular attention must be paid to incentives in this regard, just as Sears had to pay attention to its incentives program for car repair advisors when it discovered that some advisors might have recommended unnecessary repairs. Are there incentives that would bring employees honor and fame but would harm individual patients or, more likely, the already divided health care environment? John Griffith makes us worry about this problem when he explores the detailed cases of health care management ethics gone awry.

Thus health care management ethics includes the ability to conduct an open discussion of the values that should be embodied in the institution and its public actions. This discussion can lead to the development of ideas and contributions that help make the individual part of the health care delivery team. More importantly, it can benefit the employees by helping them develop their own sense of moral commitments and conscience. Perhaps the manager could establish programs that reward the development of the human and humane qualities of all employees, so that the entire organization, not just the caregivers, exemplifies compassion for the sick and debilitated. Such programs might include career training, not only in one's field but also in values clarification and development, and individual enhancement as a person. In this way, the executive could be satisfied that the highest forms of human development are part of his or her own stature as a manager, as well as part of the institutional conscience that is carried out in the mission and philosophy.

Most managers are reluctant to fix anything before a problem occurs, understandably preferring to address the myriad of current problems and challenges that beset every institution. This tendency is analogous to the tendency in modern medicine to prefer intervention to prevention. In the end, more damage is done by not anticipating and addressing potential problems. Ethical standards of practice do not just happen automatically. They require explicit attention, articulation, education, practice, reinforcement, and rewards.

Fourth, what are the obligations to the institution? The health care organization itself must be managed with consistently high ethical and professional standards. This means that the health care executive, acting with other appropriate responsible parties, must ensure an environment conducive for carrying out the task of quality health care and for accomplishing the mission, philosophy, and goals of the individual institution.

John Griffith suggests that building an ethics consensus is the role-specific duty of health care managers. While consensus ethics appeals to administrative interests, since it satisfies the most individuals and the most competing interests while protecting the institution's and the patients well-being, it might not properly respect the importance of acting on principle, with which Griffith begins his discussion of health care management ethics. Sometimes, not always of course, but sometimes, the right and good thing to do is supported by a minority. We are all familiar with the ethical curmudgeon who refuses to go along with the crowd. Sometimes such persons are blustery and pompous. But at other times, their insights need protection from the vacuousness of a group consensus if the latter is not properly developed and reflects a majority rule rather than a consensus. While trying to achieve consensus, then, managers should always be wary of the pitfalls of too many people thinking alike.

These difficult responsibilities can best be implemented in an environment in which all employees are encouraged to develop their standards of ethics and care to the fullest, by calling forth from them their highest moral commitments. Needless to say this cannot be done without attention to all the features of health care ethics, particularly those that stress the moral character of the executive and of the institution itself.

Fifth, what are the manager's social obligations? This question brings us back to the difficulties noted at the beginning of this foreword. There is a decided requirement that health care executives include themselves in the national debate about health care reform.

A national consensus is building for reform of the health care system—with good reason. Virtually alone among advanced countries, the United States does not yet consider it a right for all citizens to have equal access to health care. At the very least, coverage for basic health care for all is a desirable goal. It is not just unfortunate that millions of us have no access to health care and that the middle class often can no longer afford it. Rather it is unjust, since not providing it has been an act of political will.

Nonetheless, reform stems from two competing interests. Some support for reform arises from high-minded principles of justice while other support stems from a desire to control costs that rise annually at twice the rate of inflation. Many countries have been able to combine both interests in reasonable plans, but it is difficult. How can we simultaneously provide greater coverage at less cost? If we do not succeed, our products become even less competitive on the world market.

The issue lay confined to academic discussion until voters made their concerns known. Presidential candidates are now touting their own version of such reform, as are senators and congressmen and -women. In the midst of the politics it is too easy to forget that health care is a good and a service prerequisite for the well-being of all human beings.

In earlier times the essential moral quality of health care was embedded in the professional codes of the caregivers themselves, largely physicians and nurses. With the rise of modern, technological health care, the former one-on-one relationship between doctor and patient became institutionalized. Hospitals were no longer like a hotel where physicians signed their patients in and out at will. Suddenly, with escalating costs and the subsequent social and political monitoring, the doctor-patient relationship became a provider-patient one, with government, third party payers, institutions themselves, and many other specialists and ancillary caregivers counted as well. All of these players have complementary and sometimes competing interests in the reform of the health system.

Such a radical transformation of the original doctor-patient relationship creates a sense of chaos and a loss of control, especially over essential values in caring for individuals in our society. There are some overriding ethical considerations in the design of any national health program. The first must be that the patients ought to be able to control their care so they do not experience difficulties and delays in obtaining appropriate and approved treatment. The second is that the moral character of the health delivery institutions and of the health care practitioners is not destroyed through bureaucratic requirements. The third ethical consideration is that, since some form of rationing will be required regarding specific treatments to be made available, the national health program itself should be designed to be as efficient as possible. This consideration means that greater effort must be made than has been made yet to put available monies in patient care rather than in administrative overhead costs. Fourth, the quality of human judgment and flexibility for treating individual differences should be maintained as far as possible, so that formulaic responses to human pain and misery are avoided. Otherwise, treating people with respect will diminish.

Modern health care is a unique melding of charity and business, of compassion and attention to fiscal responsibility. If health care institutions are required to maintain this delicate balance, so too should the national health program that emerges from political debate. Incentives to hold down costs and to increase the quality of care should be built into the plan. But so too should incentives to cooperate rather than compete, to ensure commitment to patients and their values as well as the survival of institutions. No institution should benefit by shunning essential care. Sharing the burden of expensive and unreimbursed care among institutions ought also to be designed into the national health program. This sharing will still be required since not all health care interventions will be covered under any conceivable program.

Health care institutions can be said to have a conscience. This term is a convenient shorthand for the sum total of their mission and commitments. Individuals within institutions, including the doctors practicing there, should have a say in the formation of the mission and values of the institution, and should commit themselves to those values. If administrators try to arrange for the care of individuals without health care insurance, then the doctors with admitting privileges might be asked to help. If they refuse, should they be allowed to continue to have such privileges if their refusal violates a commitment of the institution and its leaders and staff?

Executives and staff ought to discuss and formulate policy positions, so that they can contribute to the national debate about the outline, design, and implementation of a national health program. Some questions might be, if basic care is to be provided, what would not be covered? What sort of rationing plan would be the most just? Should there be rationing? If so, can the public be urged to discuss different proposals for rationing that might be considered just? Should not one's own institution be part of that public discussion? What leadership might it provide?

These are not just strategic questions. They represent the moral center of the enterprise that is health care delivery.

This book is suffused with a love of the profession of health care management. From his experience and leadership, John Griffith is able to offer much more than most others have done for our ethical reflection. Now is the time to read and reflect. For the challenges of the future will certainly not diminish their assault on the moral character of the leaders in health care institution.

> David C. Thomasma, Ph.D.
> The Fr. Michael I. English, S. J.
>   Professor of Medical Ethics
>   Director: Medical Humanities Program
>   Loyola University of Chicago Medical Center

Preface

This book arises from a love of the profession of health care management, some painful personal contact with its moral challenges, and a recognition that those challenges are rarely illustrated or articulated. It is offered with considerable humility, in the belief that well-intentioned managers can improve their ethical perceptiveness and responsiveness by reading it and thinking about the issues it raises.

It might be said that I rebounded into the profession. I grew up in a hospital administrator's home, but I tentatively examined several other careers for myself. One summer in the manufacturing sector, making soap, was enough to convince me that health care offers unique personal rewards. I have never regretted that decision. There is an intrinsic satisfaction in providing people with health service, and a manager has an opportunity to work on a scale no individual practitioner can reach. The question, Why am I doing this? always has an answer at some level: Because it helps people with things they really need.

I hold that conviction as firmly today as I did in 1955. Despite the almost unbelievable complexity—I work now with abstractions of abstractions, many steps removed from the patient's side—it is not hard to remember that there are real people whose life cycle is profoundly affected by what I can and cannot do. It seems to me that pain and suffering will be tangibly reduced if I do a good job. The book is an effort to make clear how that is true, in the hopes that it will itself contribute but also that it will help others gain the satisfaction I have gained.

With the satisfaction of doing a good job comes the pain of a poor one. Over 35 years, I have had the chance not only to fail and see the painful results of my own failure but to see the problems encountered by others more closely than I would ever have chosen. The book arises in part from some of these failures. It deliberately uses them as cases in an effort to focus as many readers as possible on the dynamics of how good people and good systems can go awry. In so doing, perhaps we can prevent similar failings.

Some of the most dedicated and most respected organizations in the health care field are painfully exposed in these cases. No one is more sorry than I that this is so. The question will certainly be asked why it is useful to rake over this unfortunate history. I believe the answer is that we—the profession as a whole—really do these things and that it is only by recognition and acceptance of our failings that we can improve. The problems reflected here are universal. The cases and the institutions involved differ only a small degree from what occurs daily and inevitably in our field. In fact, efforts to cover up our transgressions underlie several of the cases, and in the long run, they represent denials of the moral challenge.

I hope the book will illustrate that the moral challenges of management are significantly different from those of the clinical professions. Our task is not so much to decide the complex questions of modern medical ethics as to establish systems that help them decide. The book does not dwell on the subject matter of medical ethics itself not only because there are many excellent books on the subject but also because those books do not answer the problems raised by the cases in this book.

Whether the book will really help health care managers improve their behavior will probably never be known. There are those who say that ethics cannot be taught at this level. "Telling right from wrong... is not all that hard; the hard part is overcoming laziness and cowardice to do what one perfectly well knows one should."[1] I disagree.[2] At least in our field, it is not necessarily easy to tell right from wrong. And more to the point, building systems to help people do what they should is the essence of management. Combatting "laziness and cowardice," or less theatrically helping people to do their best by providing them with tools, systems, reports, and incentives, is what management is all about. People can learn and can be taught to be better managers. The book is dedicated to the premise that they can learn to be more moral managers.

John R. Griffith

Notes

1. M. Levin, "Ethics Courses: Useless," *New York Times*, 25 November 1989, op-ed.
2. The Hastings Center, *The Teaching of Ethics in Higher Education* (Hastings-on-Hudson, NY: The Center, 1980).

Acknowledgments

Two very different acknowledgments are important to this book.

The first is to the three institutions—the Bethesda Naval Hospital; St. Elizabeth's of Dayton, Ohio; and Blue Cross and Blue Shield of Michigan—whose unfortunate histories have become cases to improve our futures. They have not given and were not asked to give consent or approval of the cases, which are entirely the work of the authors noted. They did, however, graciously contribute the information used in the epilogues in Part IV. Those contributions strengthen that part in several ways, and they were virtuous acts in the spirit of the moral challenge.

The second is to my teachers in ethics. As will soon become clear, I am not an ethicist or philosopher by training. What little I have been able to incorporate into this book comes from the sources I have tried to cite appropriately. I am particularly grateful to William K. Frankena, whose succinct summary *Ethics* provided most of the outline of the book and helped form the early chapters, and also to David C. Thomasma, whose patient reading and thoughtful criticism helped me clarify and support the commentaries of Parts III and IV.

Suggested Readings

Part I

Frankena, W. K. *Ethics.* 2d ed. New York: Prentice-Hall, 1973.

Part II

Beauchamp, T. *Ethics Theory and Business.* Englewood Cliffs, NJ: Prentice-Hall, 1979.

Part III

Graber, G. C., and D. C. Thomasma. *Theory and Practice in Medical Ethics.* New York: Continuum Publishing, 1989.

Hastings Center Report. Published six times annually. Briarcliff Manor, NY: Hastings Center.

Part IV

McIntyre, A. *After Virtue: A Study in Moral Theory.* 2d ed. Notre Dame, IN: University of Notre Dame Press, 1984.

———. *Ethics at Work.* Boston: Harvard Business Review Paperback, Harvard University, 1991.

Part I

Introduction

Ethical Commitments of Health Care Managers

> Act so as to treat humanity always as an end and never only as a means.
> —Immanuel Kant

Humanity as an End

This book assumes Kant's imperative. It accepts as a starting point that the moral challenge of health care managers is to see that the portion of the health care system under our control "treat[s] humanity always as an end" and to influence the rest of the world insofar as possible to do likewise. The opportunities are endless, not only in our personal behavior, where we can each respond with more humanity to the individuals we face, but through our organizations, where if we are skillful as managers, we increase the ability of others to be more humane toward patients, families, and co-workers. This goal is not trivial or superficial. Humanity is too scarce in the world to overlook even the smallest opportunity to make it an end. In health care more than other activities, we deal with such critical and fundamental issues of life that the core of our business must be the loving outreach of one human to another, the very essence of the word *humanity*.

The challenge presents itself to managers as a continuous series of individual tests that are often difficult enough to frighten beginners and perplex the most accomplished. Any manager can expect to fail some of these tests but also to succeed and in that success to gain great personal satisfaction and collegial recognition. Increasing the extent to which humanity is truly an end is one of the central rewards of any vocation. The extraordinary opportunity to do so in health care management is one item on the small list of distinctions that demarcates health care management both from management in other fields and from the more directly healing professions.

Like with many other aspects of health care management, the moral challenges are frequently underrated by, and sometimes invisible to those who are not themselves members of our small profession. The doctors, nurses, and trustees with whom we work daily, let alone our spouses and friends, can be expected to see the challenges differently, dimly, or not at all. There are many recent, well-regarded books on medical ethics that define the major recurring moral questions in terms of the response of individual practitioners to individual patients. None considers the central question of management, How do we structure the intercourse of people so that organizations encourage individuals to make the moral response, so that as frequently as possible, humanity is served as an end?

The word *humanity* itself opens an avenue to understanding the moral challenge of health care management. It immediately implies extension beyond individual patients to include family and friends of the sick, co-workers, and the community at large. Kant's term suggests an emphasis on people as a whole, consistent with the breadth of management responsibility.

The phrase also suggests more than just *life* as an end. The word *humanity* implies dimensions of meaning, value, and satisfaction that carry it beyond biological existence alone. Its breadth captures the essence of such concepts as the World Health Organization definition of *health,*

> a state of complete physical, social, emotional, and spiritual well-being and not merely the absence of disease and infirmity [1]

the American Hospital Association's (AHA's) "Ethical Conduct for Health Care Institutions,"

> ...institutions should be concerned with the overall health status of their communities....[2]

and the American College of Healthcare Executives' "Code of Ethics,"

> The fundamental objectives of the healthcare management profession are to enhance the overall quality of life, dignity and well-being of every individual needing healthcare services; and to create a more equitable, accessible, effective and efficient healthcare system.[3]

Kant's maxim is an insightful summary of much previous thought in the Judeo-Christian tradition. It might be only a restatement of

Christ's admonition, "Do unto others as you would have others do unto you."[4] It follows well the one-sentence precis of the Torah attributed to Maimonides, "That which you would not welcome yourself, you must not do to your fellow man." (He is alleged to have added, "The rest is commentary.") It is also summarizes one of the major secular rules of ethical behavior, called *universalization*. Universalization requires that any action be tested for fairness by examining its appropriateness to different or opposite sets of individuals, for example by reversing the parties of the action or substituting groups of people with different social or economic status.

Kant's doctrine is clearly among the most popular ideas of western civilization, but there are alternatives and even disputes. Certain religions emphasize the subordinance of man to God, in effect rephrasing the imperative as, "humanity as an end *as God wills it to be*." Some religious health care institutions emphasize the primacy of God's will in their missions and actions. This emphasis does not necessarily create cause for dispute. Even the strictest reading of religious principle accepts much of the Kantian approach, and most of this book applies with slight modification. Public and not-for-profit organizations avoid the reference to God's will as a matter of policy, implementing the freedom of religion concept from the Bill of Rights.

Somewhat more difficult are the concepts of moral superiority sometimes ascribed to Nietzsche. These concepts involve a judgment about the moral superiority or worth of one human being over another. The more extreme forms, such as the concept of the superiority of the white race, the eugenics movement of the early twentieth century,[5] and Hitler's final solution to the Jewish problem, are now unacceptable even as ideas for discussion. It is important to note that these ideas had surprising popular support for brief periods in history, and others like them form a more or less constant theme of human xenophobia. Lesser forms of superiority theories have had their impact on the U.S. health care system. In particular, a belief in the importance of helping the worthy victim in the nineteenth century led to focusing America's hospitals on short-term illnesses of people who could be expected to return to work.[6] The result, diminished attention to mental and chronic disease, is still with us. In the twentieth and twenty-first centuries, the concept of judging the worth of humans appears and will appear in the debates and decisions regarding AIDS care, substance abuse, and priorities for organ transplants. It might underlie more of the current situation, with 30,000,000 Americans without health insurance, than many of us would like to admit.

6 Introduction

The common theme of these approaches is the identification of a superior and an inferior group. Kant's imperative (and Christ's[7]) precludes judging the worth of different individuals, including of course, different recipients or providers of health care. There are probably two main arguments for a universal, nonjudgmental stance:

1. God may reward you for it, or it might simply be the right thing to do. The themes of mercy, love, and charity run through all the Judeo-Christian tradition. "[T]hou shalt love thy neighbor as thyself," and "Judge not, that ye be not judged," are useful summaries.[8]
2. It can be very practical, either because you might yourself somehow fall into the victimized group or because they might revolt.

Despite the popularity of "humanity as an end," history is a record of humanity's difficulties in achieving it. The health care system of the United States is no exception. With its burdensome costs, uneven access, variable outcomes, and large discrepancies in provider status and incomes, it is a patchwork of triumphs and failures. In many of its failures, patients, employees, and bystanders are to some extent exploited as means.

Health care managers have opportunities to treat humanity as an end each time we act to improve the efficiency, quality, and effectiveness of our organizations. The moral challenge of management is in overcoming the forces that limit the achievement of Kant's ideal, changing the pattern so that triumphs are greater and failures are fewer. It is a challenge that is intrinsic in the practice of the health care management profession, that will not cease, and that can never be safely overlooked. There will never be enough resources or time to find and treat the last measure of need. There will always be conflicting views on the definition of the end and the means. No matter how much technology advances, there will always be an end to life and therefore a frontier to the contribution health care can make.

About This Book

This book is about the moral challenge for health care managers, how to understand it, accept it, and perhaps improve your success. It accepts sincerely and completely both Kant's imperative and the painstaking efforts of colleagues at the AHA and ACHE that resulted in their statements of ethical obligation. (They are reprinted in full in Appendixes I.A and I.B at the end of Part I.)

The book has three additional parts. Each consists of a few cases, very brief commentaries on the cases designed to stimulate careful, thoughtful review, and an essay on some of the implications that follow from the cases. Part II is a discussion of the origins of ethical beliefs, or theories of moral obligation, and their impact on modern health care management. A theory of moral obligation is a framework of belief that an individual can use to guide specific actions. Each of us must have a personal theory to handle the multiple decisions with ethical consequences we face each day.

Understanding the origins of theories of moral obligations is important for two reasons. First, it helps us extend and strengthen our personal theories. Understanding the sources of our beliefs and examining their consequences helps us remember them and apply them more consistently as opportunities arise. Second, it shows the alternatives that are available to deal with conflicting theories. Most of us have theories that are similar but not identical to the popular consensus. Although Americans share many beliefs, we diverge at several key points in our theories of moral obligation. The freedom of individuals to follow their own moral theories is deeply imbedded in the U.S. Constitution and in judicial law. Like freedom of religion, it is generally accepted in an ethical sense as well. That is, it is part of most of our personal theories of obligation. However, the few moral theory conflicts that arise in health care tend to occur on the most fundamental issues and can easily become destructive. A health care manager's moral challenge includes understanding where people's moral views may differ and how these conflicts can be handled.

Part III is a discussion of ethical dilemmas that arise within a consistent theory of obligations. The theory the book follows is an expansion of Kant's imperative. It is a widespread one, a set of beliefs consistent with utilitarian values, applied with beneficence and justice toward one's fellow human beings. Ethical dilemmas arise when there are several moral obligations that cannot all be honored (called conflicting *prima facie* obligations). The conflicting obligations must be rank-ordered and the lesser-ranked obligations sacrificed.

Conflicting *prima facie* obligations occur routinely in such matters as the need for health care workers to have time off versus the need of patients to have safe treatment or the need for profit versus the need for charitable care. They can also arise in designing decision processes, like in the need for prompt, decisive response versus the need for participation and discussion. And they are inescapably with us in some of the major policy questions of the day: Is it better to sustain the old or prevent illness in newborns, better to give the transplant organ to patient A or patient B, better to continue the apparently successful clinical trial or to stop it, better to make care of the poor more equitable or extend the frontier for the paying majority.

(There are those who would argue that the answer to these questions is morally obvious; by their theory of moral obligations there is no conflict. To these arguments there are three responses: (1) Under the theories of moral obligations that most of us have, the answers are not so clear. (2) The daily newspaper or any other record of history shows that the implementation of any theory is likely to be difficult. The obligation of managers extends to implementation as well. (3) It is easy to be lulled by an incomplete theory. Many times there are real cases that destroy an apparently universal rule.)

Health care managers, with their commitments to respecting the ethical values of others and to extending their own and their organization's goals for beneficence, find themselves constantly weighing conflicting obligations. The process of selection among them is often a strenuous challenge. The choices can be personally painful. Selections can cause grave difficulties in a very practical sense. Bystanders with different values or just different perspectives are quick to criticize, even if they are slow to accept the responsibility to decide. Difficulties with conflicting *prima facie* obligations underlie many unplanned resignations of health care managers.

Just like with other aspects of management decision making, there are rules and procedures to improve the handling of conflicting *prima facie* obligations. These apply both to the actions of the manager and to the design of the decision processes of the organization. They are discussed in Part III.

Part IV deals with the extent to which organizations per se, as opposed to their members as individuals, can promote humanity as an end. Is it possible to design bureaucratic systems in ways that increase the chance that humanity is treated as an end in all the actions that make up modern health care? If it is possible, is it practical in this era of economic competition? These questions lead to considering how managers can enhance their personal ability to treat humanity as an end and how they can enhance the ability of other individuals in the organization. The exercise of influence over other individuals itself raises an ethical question that is central to management: the right of managers to command and the impact of command on moral behavior. These are questions of moral virtue, that is, of the goodness of individuals, extended to the level of the organization.

There is a good deal of accumulated wisdom about virtue, how to be a good person and to remain a good person in the face of challenges. It is clear that some individuals are more virtuous—that is, more sensitive to humanity as an end—than others and arguable that individuals can improve their virtue by faith, hard work, and self-control. To what extent can the same be said for hospitals, clinics, aged care programs, and health insurance companies? Can those organizations make individuals more virtuous, at least in their capacities as agents for the corporation? The chapter begins by exploring how managers can promote virtue in themselves. It then explores the evidence that the manager can favorably influence moral behavior of others in the organization, that certain management styles and practices promote good moral (as well as practical) decisions while others encourage cynicism and reduce the achievement of the ends of humanity. We will discuss how this evidence relates to how managers can promote virtue in health care organizations.

Each of these three chapters begins with a selection of cases that illustrate the moral challenges involved. The cases have no right answers, but they raise a series of moral questions that are also important management considerations. Although some of these questions are identified in a brief commentary, the wise reader will want to think independently about what these questions are. He or she might then turn to the essay concluding the chapter to gain the ideas of others before considering how a solution might be designed and implemented in a real management environment.

Notes

1. "Declaration of Alma-Ata," in *Primary Health Care*, Report of the International Conference on Primary Health Care (Geneva, Switzerland: World Health Organization, 1978), 2.
2. American Hospital Association, *Ethical Conduct for Health Care Institutions*, management advisory, American Hospital Association, Chicago, IL.
3. The American College of Healthcare Executives, *Code of Ethics*, American College of Healthcare Executives, Chicago, IL.
4. Golden Rule, common paraphrase of Matthew 7:12 and Luke 6:31.

5. R. F. Chadwick, ed., *Ethics, Reproduction, and Genetic Control* (London: Croom Helm, 1987).
6. C. E. Rosenberg, *The Care of Strangers: The Rise of America's Hospital System* (New York: Basic Books, 1987).
7. "Inasmuch as ye have done it unto one of the least of these my brethren, ye have done it unto me." Matthew 25:40.
8. Leviticus 19:18; Matthew 7:1.

Appendix I.A

American College of Healthcare Executives

Code of Ethics

Preamble

The purpose of the Code of Ethics of the American College of Healthcare Executives is to serve as a guide to conduct for affiliates. It contains standards of ethical behavior for healthcare executives in their professional relationships. These relationships include members of the healthcare executive's organization and other organizations. Also included are patients or others served, colleagues, the community and society as a whole. The Code of Ethics also incorporates standards of ethical behavior governing personal behavior, particularly when that conduct directly relates to the role and identity of the healthcare executive.

The fundamental objectives of the healthcare management profession are to enhance overall quality of life, dignity and well-being of every individual needing healthcare services; and to create a more equitable, accessible, effective and efficient healthcare system.

Healthcare executives have an obligation to act in ways that will merit the trust, confidence and respect of healthcare professionals and

---

As amended by the Council of Regents at its annual meeting on July 28, 1992.

Reprinted with the permission of the American College of Healthcare Executives, Chicago, Illinois.

the general public. To do so, healthcare executives must lead lives that embody an exemplary system of values and ethics.

In fulfilling their commitments and obligations to patients or others served, healthcare executives function as moral agents. Since every management decision affects the health and well-being of both individuals and communities, healthcare executives must evaluate the possible outcomes of their decisions and accept full responsibility for the consequences. In organizations that deliver healthcare services, they must safeguard and foster the rights, interests and prerogatives of patients or others served. The role of moral agent requires that healthcare executives speak out and take actions necessary to promote such rights, interests and prerogatives if they are threatened.

I. The Healthcare Executive's Responsibilities to the Profession of Healthcare Management

The healthcare executive shall:

A. Uphold the values, ethics and mission of the healthcare management profession;

B. Conduct all personal and professional activities with honesty, integrity, respect, fairness and good faith in a manner that will reflect well upon the profession;

C. Comply with all laws in the jurisdictions in which the healthcare executive is located, or conducts professional or personal activities;

D. Maintain competence and proficiency in healthcare management by implementing a personal program of assessment and continuing professional education;

E. Avoid the exploitation of professional relationships for personal gain;

F. Use this code to further the interests of the profession and not for selfish reasons;

G. Respect professional confidences;

H. Enhance the dignity and image of the healthcare management profession through positive public information programs;

I. Refrain from participating in any endorsement or publicity that demeans the credibility and dignity of the healthcare management profession; and

ACHE Code of Ethics

J. Refrain from using the College's credential or affiliation with the College to promote or endorse external commercial products or services.

II. The Healthcare Executive's Obligations to Patients or Others Served, to the Organization and to Employees

A. Commitments to patients or others served

  The healthcare executive shall:

  1. Assure the existence of a process to evaluate the quality of care or service rendered;
  2. Avoid exploitation of relationships for personal advantage;
  3. Avoid practicing or facilitating discrimination and institute safeguards to prevent discriminatory organizational practices;
  4. Assure the existence of a process that will advise patients or others served of the rights, opportunities, responsibilities and risks regarding available healthcare services;
  5. Provide a process that assures the autonomy and self-determination of patients or others served; and
  6. Assure the existence of procedures that will safeguard the confidentiality and privacy of patients or others served.

B. Commitments to the organization

  The healthcare executive shall:

  1. Provide healthcare services consistent with available resources and assure the existence of a resource allocation process that considers ethical ramifications;
  2. Conduct both competitive and cooperative activities in ways that improve community healthcare services;
  3. Lead the organization in the use and improvement of standards of management and sound business practices;
  4. Respect the customs and practices of patients or others served, consistent with the organization's philosophy; and
  5. Be truthful in all forms of professional and organizational

communication and avoid information that is false, misleading, and deceptive or information that would create unreasonable expectations.

C. Responsibilities to employees

Healthcare executives have an ethical and professional obligation to employees of the organizations they manage that encompass but are not limited to:

1. Creating a working environment conducive for underscoring employee ethical conduct and behavior.
2. Assuring that individuals may freely express ethical concerns and providing mechanisms for discussing and addressing such concerns.
3. Assuring a working environment that is free from harassment, sexual and other; coercion of any kind, especially to perform illegal or unethical acts; and discrimination on the basis of race, creed, color, sex, ethnic origin, age or disability.
4. Assuring a working environment that is conducive to proper utilization of employees' skills and abilities.
5. Paying particular attention to the employee's work environment and job safety.
6. Establishing appropriate grievance and appeals mechanisms.

III. Conflicts of Interest

A conflict of interest may be only a matter of degree, but exists when the healthcare executive:

A. Is in a position to benefit directly or indirectly by using authority or inside information, or allows a friend, relative or associate to benefit from such authority or information.
B. Uses authority or information to make a decision to intentionally affect the organization in an adverse manner.

The healthcare executive shall:

A. Conduct all personal and professional relationships in such a way that all those affected are assured that management decisions are made in the best interests of the organization and the individuals served by it;

B. Disclose to the appropriate authority any direct or indirect financial or personal interests that might pose potential conflicts of interest;
C. Accept no gifts or benefits offered with the expectation of influencing a management decision; and
D. Inform the appropriate authority and other involved parties of potential conflicts of interest related to appointments or elections to boards or committees inside or outside the healthcare executive's organization.

IV. The Healthcare Executive's Responsibilities to Community and Society

The healthcare executive shall:

A. Work to identify and meet the healthcare needs of the community;
B. Work to assure that all people have reasonable access to healthcare services;
C. Participate in public dialogue on healthcare policy issues and advocate solutions that will improve health status and promote quality healthcare;
D. Consider the short-term and long-term impact of management decisions on both the community and on society; and
E. Provide prospective consumers with adequate and accurate information, enabling them to make enlightened judgments and decisions regarding services.

V. The Healthcare Executive's Duty to Report Violations of the Code

An affiliate of the College who has reasonable grounds to believe that another affiliate has violated this Code has a duty to communicate such facts to the Ethics Committee.

Ethical Policy Statement: Impaired Healthcare Executives

Statement of the Problem

The American College of Healthcare Executives recognizes that impairment in the form of alcoholism, substance abuse, chemical dependency, mental/emotional instability or senility is a problem that affects all of society. Nineteen percent of Americans have used illicit drugs and/or are classified as alcoholics, according to the Alcohol and Drug Abuse Administration. Substance abuse is a pervasive problem in today's society, affecting individuals of all ages and in all walks of life. Mental/emotional instability and senility are also problems that cross all boundaries in society. Studies by the National Institute of Mental Health indicate that 22% of Americans are thought to experience some kind of mental disorder over their lifetime.

Impaired healthcare executives affect not only themselves and their families, but they also have a significant impact on their profession; their professional society; their organizations, colleagues, patients, clients, and others served; their communities; and society as a whole. Impairment typically leads to misconduct in the form of incompetence and unsafe or unprofessional behavior, which can also lead to substantial costs associated with loss of productivity and errors in judgment.

The impaired healthcare executive can damage the public image of his or her organization of employment. Public confidence in the organization diminishes if it appears that the organization is not being managed with consistently high standards of professional and ethical practice. This lack of public confidence may cause the community to deem the organization unworthy of its support.

Society expects healthcare executives to practice the standards of good health that they advocate for the public. Impaired healthcare executives diminish the credibility of the profession and its ability to

---

Approved by the Board of Governors of the American College of Healthcare Executives on February 11, 1991.

Reprinted with the permission of the American College of Healthcare Executives, Chicago, Illinois.

manage society's healthcare when they are not appropriately managing their own personal health.

Policy Position

The preamble of the American College of Healthcare Executives Code of Ethics states that "healthcare executives have an obligation to act in ways that will merit the trust, confidence and respect of healthcare professionals and the general public. To do this, healthcare executives must lead lives that embody an exemplary system of values and ethics."

The American College of Healthcare Executives believes that all healthcare executives have an ethical and a professional obligation to:

- Maintain a personal health status that is free from impairment.
- Refrain from all professional activities if impaired.
- Expeditiously seek a cure if impairment occurs.
- Urge impaired colleagues to expeditiously seek a cure and to refrain from all professional activities while impaired.
- Report the impairment to the appropriate person or persons, should the colleague refuse to seek professional assistance and should the state of impairment persist.
- Recommend or provide, within one's employing organization, avenues for reporting impairment and either access or referral to treatment or assistance programs.
- Urge the community to provide information and resources for assistance and treatment of alcoholism, substance abuse, mental/emotional instability, and senility as needed and appropriate.

Appendix I.B

American Hospital Association

Ethical Conduct for Health Care Institutions

Introduction

Health care institutions, by virtue of their roles as health care providers, employers, and community health resources, have special responsibilities for ethical conduct and practices. Their broad range of patient care, education, public health, social service, and business functions is essential to the health and well-being of their communities. In general, the public expects that they will conduct themselves in an ethical manner that emphasizes a basic community service orientation.

This management advisory is intended to assist members of the American Hospital Association to better define the ethical aspects and implications of institutional policies and practices. It is offered with the understanding that individual decisions seldom reflect an absolute ethical right or wrong, and that each institution's leadership in making policy and decisions must take into account the needs and values of the institution, its medical community, and employees and those of individual patients, their families, and the community as a whole.

Reprinted with permission of the American Hospital Association, copyright 1990.

This management advisory was reaffirmed by the Institutional Practices Committee in 1990, was developed by the AHA Technical Panel on Biomedical Ethics, and was initially approved by the Board of Trustees in 1987.

The governing board of the institution is responsible for establishing and periodically evaluating the ethical standards that guide institutional practices. The chief executive officer is responsible for assuring that hospital medical staff, employees, and volunteers and auxilians understand and adhere to these standards and for promoting an environment sensitive to differing values and conducive to ethical behavior.

This management advisory examines the hospital's ethical responsibilities to its community and patients as well as those deriving from its organizational roles as employer and a business entity. Although some responsibilities also may be included in legal and accreditation requirements, it should be remembered that legal, accreditation, and ethical obligations often overlap and that ethical obligations often extend beyond legal and accreditation requirements.

Community Role

- Health care institutions should be concerned with the overall health status of their communities while continuing to provide direct patient services. This principle requires them to communicate and work with other health care and social agencies to improve the availability and provision of health promotion and education and services as well as patient care and to take a leadership role in enhancing public health and continuity of care in the community.
- Health care institutions are responsible for fair and effective use of available health care delivery resources to promote access to comprehensive and affordable health care services of high quality. This responsibility extends beyond the resources of the given institution to include efforts to coordinate with other health care providers and to share in community solutions for providing care for the medically indigent and others.
- All health care institutions have community service responsibilities which may include care for the poor and the uninsured, provision of needed services, and education and various programs designed to meet the specific needs of their communities. Not-for-profit institutions, in consideration of their community service origins, Hill-Burton obligations, and tax status, should be particularly sensitive to the importance of providing and designing services for their communities.

- Health care institutions, being dependent upon community confidence and support, are accountable to the public, and therefore their communications and disclosure of information and data related to the institution should be clear, accurate, and sufficiently complete to assure that it is not misleading. Such disclosure should be aimed primarily at better public understanding of health issues, the services available to prevent and treat illness, and patients' rights and responsibilities relating to health care decisions.
- As health care institutions operate in an increasingly competitive environment, they should consider the overall welfare of their communities and their own missions in determining their activities, service mixes, and business ventures and conduct their business activities in an ethical manner.

Patient Care

- Health care institutions are responsible for assuring that the care provided to each patient is appropriate and of the highest quality they are able to provide. Health care institutions should establish and follow procedures to verify the credentials of physicians and other health professionals, assess and improve quality of care, and review appropriateness of utilization.
- Health care institutions should have policies and practices that support the process of informed consent for diagnostic and therapeutic procedures and that respect and promote the patient's responsibility for decision making.
- Health care institutions are responsible for assuring confidentiality of patient-specific information. They are responsible for providing safeguards to prevent unauthorized release of information and establishing procedures for authorizing release of data.
- Health care institutions should assure that the psychological, social, spiritual, and physical needs and cultural beliefs and practices of patients and families are recognized and should promote employee and medical staff sensitivity to the full range of such needs and practices.
- Health care institutions should assure respect for and reasonable accommodation of individual religious and social beliefs and customs of patients whenever possible.

- Health care institutions should have specific mechanisms or procedures to resolve conflicting values and ethical dilemmas among patients, their families, medical staff, employees, the institution, and the community.

Organizational Conduct

- The policies and practices of health care institutions should respect the professional ethical codes and responsibilities of their employees and medical staff members and be sensitive to institutional decisions that employees might interpret as compromising their ability to provide high-quality health care.
- Health care institutions should have policies and practices that provide for equitably-administered employee policies and practices.
- To the extent possible and consistent with the ethical commitments of the institution, health care institutions should accommodate the desires of employees and medical staff to embody religious and moral values in their professional activities.
- Health care institutions should have written policies on conflict of interest that apply to officers, governing board members, physicians, and others who make or influence decisions for or on behalf of the institution. These policies should recognize that individuals in decision-making or administrative positions often have duality of interests that may not ordinarily present conflicts. But they should provide mechanisms for identifying and addressing conflicts when they do exist.
- Health care institutions should communicate their mission, values, and priorities to the employees and volunteers, whose patient care and service activities are the most visible embodiment of the institution's ethical commitments and values.

AHA Resources

This management advisory identifies the major areas affecting the ethical conduct of health care institutions. It would be impossible for one advisory document to detail all of the factors and issues relating to each area. Additional information and guidance is available in the following AHA management advisories:

A Patient's Bill of Rights
Advertising
Discharge Planning
Disclosure of Financial and Operating Information
Disclosure of Medical Record Information
Establishment of an Employee Grievance Procedure
Ethics Committees
Imperatives of Hospital Leadership
Quality Management
Resolution of Conflicts of Interest
The Patient's Choice of Treatment Options
Verifying Physician Credentials
Verifying Credentials of Medical Students and Residents

The following AHA publications may also be useful:

Values in Conflict: Resolving Ethical Issues in Hospital Care (AHA #025002)

Effective DNR Policies: Development, Revision, and Implementation (AHA #058750)

Part II

Theories of Moral Obligation

Case 1

Abortion Policy at XYZ Community Hospital

Introductory Note: The abortion issue represents one of the most difficult situations a community health care organization can face because it reflects serious disagreement over fundamental moral questions. Although the following case is fictional, we have all heard the views expressed here, and none of us could have missed the intensity of debate in this country since *Roe v. Wade*. The case raises several questions that are a useful starting point in the discussion of health care management ethics:

1. What are the origins of the opinions so strongly held by the participants in the case, including the manager herself? Why do they believe as they do?
2. If positions on abortion can range from ardent pro-life to equally ardent pro-choice, to what extent can a secular community organization represent or advocate a specific point on the scale? What are the sources of your beliefs about the answers to these questions?
3. Could the abortion debate endanger the institution as a whole? Should this be allowed to happen? What makes you feel that it should or should not?
4. Are there better or worse ways to handle the dispute? What are the possible outcomes? Are there any that can be broadly accepted?

The case also introduces some other questions involving the appropriate behavior of the nurse and the manager, who are morally opposed to abortion. These issues will be addressed later, in Part III.

You are the administrator of a nonreligious, not-for-profit community hospital in a small city with the nearest competition about 50 miles away. *Roe v. Wade* has declared unconstitutional your state's antiabortion law, and a small group of women who are also hospital volunteers has approached you with the request that your hospital offer abortion counseling in its clinics and make its facilities available for abortion on demand. You personally have the conviction that abortion is wrong, although you have never attempted to analyze the source of your feelings or to influence the national political argument. You tell the volunteers that you will examine the feasibility of their proposal and schedule another meeting with them for one week hence.

While you are puzzling over the matter, events pass you by. Two days later the local paper carries an article reporting that your hospital is engaged in developing its policy on abortion. When you arrive at your office, the phone is ringing. The chairperson of your board tells you that a number of people have called her and that she has referred them to you and wants you to deal with them. She is unpleasantly surprised by the newspaper article, and she wants you to make a recommendation to the board on abortion policy. While the board is interested in the financial and political aspects of the situation, they also expect you to take a more philosophical point of view and present the issue in terms of what the hospital should do to be ethically correct.

Several individuals from various groups go to some lengths to deliver their views on the issue to you personally. Their views are summarized as follows:

A right-to-life representative

1. "Thou shalt not kill." It is simply wrong to kill or condone killing. Not only is this clear from the Bible, but it should be equally clearly written in the conscience of any normal human being.
2. Once you start down the primrose path, where does it end (euthanasia, killing "defectives," etc.)?

This case was prepared by Peter A. Wilson, Ph.D., and John R. Griffith.

3. Abortion will encourage immoral and irresponsible sexual conduct.

A Zero Population Growth/Planned Parenthood representative

1. The world is in danger of severe overpopulation. Every year millions starve. Anything that lowers the birth rate is desirable.
2. Unwanted children are a personal burden and usually become a social burden. They perpetuate the problems of poverty for generations.

A women's rights representative

1. Women have an absolute right to control their bodies. It is immoral to make a woman give birth to a child conceived from rape or incest or whom she cannot care for adequately.
2. This hospital is a community medical resource and should provide whenever possible whatever medical service a member of the community desires.
3. There is nothing wrong with taking human life under some circumstances. Human life is not an absolute value.

A welfare rights organization representative

1. Women will get abortions whether or not your hospital offers them. The only difference is that rich ladies will go to the hospital 50 miles down the line while poor ladies will use somebody's kitchen table.
2. We agree that human life is sacred but do not see that the issue is involved here. "Sacred" is being used to discriminate against families who already bear enough burdens. The word is a middle-class cop-out.

A doctor

1. Under many circumstances, pregnancy is disabling and as such is medically counterindicated.
2. This place is a medical resource for the community through me. I should make all the clinical judgments necessary and say how and when the hospital should be used.

Case 2

Baby Doe: Care of Severely Damaged Neonates

Introductory Note: When is it no longer appropriate to strive to maintain life? Kant's criterion of humanity becomes ambiguous as the margins of life are reached. In the Baby Doe issue, the views of a group of people who feel compelled to support the neonate's right to life as an overwhelming central objective of health care run counter to those who see it as only one of several possible goals. The question has high stakes. Many infants can be saved, some for a full life span. On the other hand, hundreds of thousands of dollars can be expended to save a single impaired life that might be a burden on the family and society as a whole. The funds could be productively employed in relieving the causes of neonatal impairment, perhaps increasing the total survival rate. And what is the right of society to impose its view on this question when it is clearly unwilling to take financial responsibility for the result?

As a result of several court suits and extensive media exposure, the federal government promulgated a very severe regulation, calling anything less than life-preserving treatment of neonates a violation of the civil rights of handicapped persons. These rules, called Baby Doe I, were overthrown by the Supreme Court in 1984. The 1985 rules, Baby Doe II, are not much less strict, although they are somewhat ambiguous:

> [The withholding of medically indicated treatments is] the failure to respond to the infant's life-threatening conditions by providing treatment (including appropriate nutrition, hydration, and medication) which, in the treating physician's (or physicians') reasonable medical judgment, will be most likely to be effective in ameliorating or correcting all such conditions, except that the term does not include the failure to provide treatment (other than appropriate nutrition, hydration, or medication)

to an infant when, in the treating physician's (or physicians') reasonable medical judgment any of the following circumstances apply: (i) The infant is chronically and irreversibly comatose (ii) The provision of such treatment would merely prolong dying, not be effective in ameliorating or correcting all of the infant's life-threatening conditions, or otherwise be futile in terms of the survival of the infant; or (iii) The provision of such treatment would be virtually futile in terms of the survival of the infant and the treatment itself under such circumstances would be inhumane.[1]

The article by Krauthammer discusses alternative criteria for deciding the individual cases, and advocates a relatively strict position. It also addresses the broader issue that underlies these debates: how we can continue as a society when honest citizens differ in apparently irreconcilable ways. Krauthammer notes that we have chosen a compromise that is "at once astonishing and sensible."[2]

Baby Doe II was successful in the sense that it took the issue out of the courts and the media, but it appears to have left a significant dissatisfaction among neonatologists who must apply the rules. A 1988 survey showed that they feel, by clear majorities, that the regulations were not necessary, interfered with parents' rights, and did not adequately deal with infant suffering. Three hypothetical cases revealed substantial difference of opinion in interpreting the regulations.[3]

The questions raised by Baby Doe are very similar to those of the abortion case. Why do people feel as they do? How does the health care organization respond? Should the highly questionable compromise be tolerated or attacked?

What To Do About 'Baby Doe'*

by Charles Krauthammer

If physicians are going to play God... let us hope they play God as God plays God.

—Paul Ramsey

---

*Reprinted from *The New Republic*, 2 September 1985, pp. 16–21, with the permission of Charles Krauthammer.

Between 1977 and 1982 a group of Oklahoma doctors conducted an experiment on children born with spina bifida. Spina bifida is a congenital malformation in which the spine does not close and is often exposed through the skin. It can lead to paralysis, retardation, and other disabilities. Before treatment became available in the early 1960s, the condition was almost universally fatal. The purpose of the experiment was to determine which spina bifida newborns to treat and which to let die. Doctors divided the infants into two groups. Those with a more favorable prognosis for a good "quality of life" were selected for immediate and aggressive treatment (surgery to close the spine, shunting water away from the brain, antibiotics). All of these babies survived. The other group of infants deemed to have a poor "quality of life" prognosis was selected for no treatment at all. Parents demanded treatment anyway for five of them, and three survived. Of the rest, all 24 died within 189 days.

This May the doctors and the hospital were threatened with a suit by groups representing the disabled and by the ACLU. The charge was discrimination against the more severely affected children. They were denied treatment because they were deemed to be not worth saving. That they were not medically beyond saving was shown by the survival of three of the five whose parents insisted on treatment even though they were chosen to die. The non-treatment decision proceeds from "a eugenic premise," writes Martin Gerry in the July issue of *Law and Medicine*, "not... that a child cannot or will not live, but... that the child should not live."

The remarkable thing about the clash between baby doctor and baby advocate—and an indication of the gulf of incomprehension that separates them—is that there was no need for daring undercover work here. The doctors published their study in the October 1983 issue of *Pediatrics*, one of their profession's leading journals. They clearly felt they had nothing to hide. The Oklahoma doctors consider what they did to be accepted, if novel, practice. The baby advocates call it euthanasia. Or, as one of their cause's most prominent propagandists, Nat Hentoff, likes to say: murder. How can reasonable people come to such wildly different conclusions?

To start with, the doctors pretend to too much reasonableness. The tone of their article, a tone of unrelieved moral flatness, seems designed to provoke indignation if not litigation. "The 'untreated survivor' has not been a significant problem in our experience," they write. "All 24 babies who have not been treated at all have died at an average of 37 days." Success. Their description of the "selection process" is casual, lacking the slightest awareness of the awful historical echoes associated with that term. And their moral calculus is so technologically streamlined that it yields results like: "Whatever decision the parents make, it is important that they be relieved of any sense of guilt." Any decision?

Still, you don't, or shouldn't, get hauled into court for transgressions of tone. You get hauled in for murder. Was this murder? There is a real question here: If we must make life-and-death decisions on behalf of others, can we ever morally choose death?

Is there a life worse than death? Judging from how adults act and talk, yes. Voluntary death is a not irrational response of people to intractable pain, or imprisonment, or dishonor, for example. (There is even a large body of opinion that would add communism to the list.) We do not assume that life is automatically the supreme value. In deciding for ourselves whether there is a life worse than death we would weigh the costs and the benefits of continued existence. But in deciding for others, as we do for a newborn, the first question is: Whose costs and whose benefits? Whose interests count: society's, the family's, or the patient's?

The societal consideration goes something like this: we are a vast society with vast needs and scarce resources. Even scarcer resources are allocated to medicine. The cost of saving and maintaining a sickly child (or adult, as Governor Richard D. Lamm of Colorado, has argued) is huge. That money could be better spent saving and sustaining many others. As Lamm put it to the elderly some years ago, at some point "we all have a duty to die" and make room for others.

This idea usually goes by the name of triage, and has almost no application to "Baby Doe" disabled newborns. For one thing, in their treatment, resources are not scarce. They are a tiny number every year, and the reason that they are not treated vigorously is to spare them or their families anguish, not to spare the country respirators. Second even if there were a shortage, it is one thing to tell the elderly to drop dead. They can weigh the invitation and choose. An infant chooses nothing. He is at our mercy. And mercy—and justice—dictate that in deciding whether he is to live or die, the federal deficit [does] not enter the calculation.

Generally, however, a different calculation is made. When families and their doctors decide not to treat a defective newborn, they are not balancing society's costs and benefits, but the family's. That includes, of course, the newborn's, but also those of the rest of the family: siblings, parents, even the "marriage" itself.

Now, these are not frivolous considerations. But they cannot be morally relevant to a decision about the life or death of a child. That idea commands a remarkable consensus in the ethical literature. The President's Commission for the Study of Ethical Problems in Medicine, for example, declares that any criteria for non-treatment must "exclude consideration of the negative effects of an impaired child's life on other persons, including parents, siblings, and society." Family members can and should be made to yield certain goods to accommodate other family members. They cannot be made to yield their lives.

In weighing life against death for a child, therefore, there is no place for the utilitarian calculations of others. It is impermissible to add the interests of society or even the family to the scale. The only standard is the child's own best interest.

Who is to represent that interest? An immediate corollary of the "child's best interest" standard is that one cannot assume that the best representative is the parents. There is a widespread assumption that parents should make unmolested life-or-death decisions for their children because they act as the child's proxy. They don't. No matter how well intentioned, parents cannot disentangle their own best interests and that of their family from that of the newborn. Nor can the doctor. He has the parents, the family, and his own profession to think of.

That is why there is a need for Big Brother, as both *The New York Times* and *The Wall Street Journal* derisively called federal intrusion into the nurseries of the country to try to prevent non-treatment of handicapped newborns.

The complaint against Big Brother usually takes three forms. First is the claim that "decisions about a child's medical care" (as the *Times* describes what was at stake in a 1983 spina bifida case on Long Island) should be left to parents and doctors. This claim rests on a linguistic sleight of hand. What is being decided in a spina bifida case is not which medical treatment is most likely to benefit the child, but whether life itself will benefit the child. Once the latter decision is made, the medical treatment is straightforward. The question is not how to preserve a life, but whether. The first is a medical question; the second, a moral one. To confuse the two is to engage in what Robert Veatch of Georgetown University's Kennedy Institute of Ethics calls "medicalizing value choices." Neither doctors nor parents, nor doctors and parents together, have a special moral sense.

A second defense of parental autonomy rests on "privacy." But in a society where child labor, child abuse, and even withholding a child from school have been deemed a legitimate concern of government, it is absurd to claim privacy for decisions about life and death.

The final defense of parental autonomy, therefore, is the notion that the parents are the child's true proxy. But it is simply false to assume that they necessarily act in the child's best interest. To ask that of a parent is to demand a rare degree of selflessness. Sainthood is not easy to mandate and it should not be the basis for policy.

That was proved dramatically in the case that started the current round of debate, the case of the Indianapolis Baby Doe. That baby was born in April 1982 with Down's syndrome and an easily correctable digestive problem. Without correction, however, the baby could not take food and would starve to death. The parents refused to order surgery. An appeals court upheld their right to make that decision. Baby Doe starved to death six days later.

Easy cases make good (moral) law. Even *The New York Times* could tell that Indianapolis Baby Doe had been wronged. In this case you could not even begin to argue that the child was allowed to die in its own best interest, in order to be spared a life of suffering. Down's syndrome babies can grow up to live rich lives. They suffer from varying degrees of retardation and some other disabilities. The extent of these, however, is wholly unpredictable at birth. As Louis Lasagna, a physician and father of a Down's syndrome child, says, their principal social disability is a "congenital inability to hate." This Baby Doe was sacrificed to the interests of others.

The "child's best interest" standard gets us partway there: it rules out deciding life or death on the basis of society's needs (triage) or on the basis of the family's. As a corollary, it rules out relying solely on parents as proxies. But saying that the surgeon general or a hospital ethics committee or a guardian *ad litem* should superintend any parental decision only opens the argument. Whoever decides, how are they to decide? What is the child's best interests?

Specifically, can it ever be death? We know from the action of sentient adults that the answer can be yes in at least two medical contexts: patients with intractable pain and patients who are dying and for whom all that medicine can offer is heroic and pointless prolongation of the process. These are easy cases. Consider a difficult case. Consider a patient who has severe spina bifida, resulting in paralysis, retardation, and recurrent medical illness. Consider, in other words, those babies in the Oklahoma experiment. What are their best interests? The President's Commission concludes that "permanent handicaps justify a decision not to provide life-sustaining treatment only when they are so severe that continued existence would not be a net benefit to the infant." "Net benefit" suggests those cost/benefit, quality-of-life considerations that the Baby Doe advocates so vociferously oppose. It sounds like a very liberal criterion. Except, adds the commission, that "the surrogate is obligated to try to evaluate benefits and burdens from the infant's own perspective."

The implications of this last condition are enormous. For adults who have known otherwise, spina bifida or some other severe disability might be considered a fate worse than death. But the child will have known nothing else. He must compare spina bifida not against normal life but against no life. If we are enjoined to make a decision from his point of view, it seems we must always choose life.

And that, argues philosopher John Arras (in an especially lucid analysis published in the April 1984 issue of the Hastings Center Report, which suggested much of this argument to me), leads to a conclusion that contradicts "moral common sense." In effect, the "child's best interest" criterion harnessed to the "child's point of view" requirement forces the following conclusion: that the only possible justification for withholding treatment is pain. There is no existence so blighted, so constricted, so isolated, so terribly cut off from human warmth or potential development that we can be induced to let it end mercifully.

This cannot be right. "Moral common sense" suggests that there is such an existence. Philosopher Richard McCormick has tried to elaborate that feeling. "Life is a relative good," he writes, "and the duty to preserve it a limited one. . . . Life is a value to be preserved only insofar as it contains some potentiality for human relationships." There are certain irreducible attributes of personhood, and if they are "simply nonexistent or would be utterly submerged or undeveloped in the mere struggle to survive, that life has achieved its potential." In other words, it is no longer worth living. It is not that "some lives are valuable, others not," say McCormick. "Of course [the individual] has, or is, a value. The only point is whether this undoubted value has any potential at all, in continuing physical survival, for attaining a share, even if reduced, in the 'higher, more important good.' "

Arras puts it more simply; there are some existences for which there do not exist "interests" to speak of. Then the "best interest" criterion itself collapses and, with it, the injunction to preserve life.

This line of reasoning contradicts the Kantian view, represented best by theologian Paul Ramsey, that "persons are not reducible to their potential." That sounds better than McCormick, I admit. But it is, I think, impossible to live with. Giving absolute primacy to life is meant to keep us from the slippery slope, but unfortunately life takes place there. If you believe that life is a divine gift, which man has no right to refuse, that is one thing. But it is difficult to accept the secular argument that no deprivation of human endowment could ever warrant the choice not to perpetuate life. If there is no relatedness, no human context for life, then it is hard to see where the "best interest" criterion is violated. I could produce (and you could imagine) a hypothetical example so awful—so awful that I cannot bring myself to write it—as to empty the "best interest" standard of any meaning.

My argument is, however, purposely hypothetical and theoretical. I don't want to be forced by Ramsey to say "never." In the extreme, it seems to me that Arras's "moral common sense" prevails. An equally important point, however, is that, practically speaking, we rarely face such extremes, even in spina bifida. Some choices are made in hell, but we don't encounter them terribly often on earth. And hardly six times a year in Oklahoma.

Even according to McCormick's criteria—a potential for relationships and development—the Oklahoma spina bifida babies did not warrant non-treatment. Since the 1960s, aggressive treatment has kept alive a large number of spina bifida children. And more than just kept alive. Only 30 percent of them are retarded. Even those with hydrocephalus, one of the conditions that apparently led the Oklahoma doctors to categorize a baby for non-treatment (though the criteria are never made explicit), have a better than 50 percent chance for being intellectually normal if they are treated reasonably early and do not develop meningitis.

The morality of the Oklahoma experiment is quite reversed. The experiment ostensibly proves that if certain severely affected patients are not treated, they will die. But before 1960 spina bifida was almost universally fatal. The proposition to be proved was already known. Moreover, the study implies that the "natural" death of those who were not treated provides retrospective moral justification for non-treatment. The experiment proves the opposite: given current technology, these were unnatural, certainly unnecessary, deaths. The experiment discredits itself.

What to do about it? All this moral talk is fine, but how can the political system possibly regulate the issue? The Reagan administration learned a rude lesson about regulating the nursery. After the Indianapolis Baby Doe case, the administration rushed out regulations requiring posted warnings in the nurseries and inviting calls to a hot line about medical neglect of impaired newborns. This led to a storm of protests from liberals (the *Times*), libertarians (the *Journal*), and doctors. Two judges agreed, and threw out two sets of Baby Doe regulations.

Then, in October 1984, Congress enacted amendments to the Child Abuse Prevention and Treatment Act that expanded the definition of "medical neglect" to include "withholding of medically indicated treatment from a disabled infant." The final regulations issued by the Department of Health and Human Services in May 1985 were less intrusive than Baby Doe I or II: we shall have smaller warning signs, hidden from general view, aimed only at medical personnel rather than passersby. But these regulations establish strict criteria for non-treatment, more Ramsey than McCormick. Treatment may be withheld only if it will prolong dying or cause too much suffering. Quality-of-life considerations are excluded. I would have preferred including them and defining them strictly (that is, "from the child's perspective"). But apparently the prevailing view was that overbroad regulations would give doctors with Oklahoma-like inclinations too much discretion. There will now be error on the side of life. We could do worse.

The strictness of these regulations is, however, mitigated by two interesting features. First, "withholding of medically indicated treatment" is recognized as a species of child abuse, and not of discrimination, as the administration had wanted. This bureaucratic distinction has serious implications. To prove discrimination you need only prove that a normal child would have received treatment. To prove child abuse you must prove that the child's own best interests were violated. The second consideration is more relevant. (If it is in the child's best interest not to be treated, so what if a nonhandicapped child might have benefited?) Furthermore, it focuses attention, albeit in veiled form, on quality of life.

The second feature is a small testimony to the ultimate wisdom of the democratic government. As Professor Thomas H. Murray points out, "given the enormous fuss"—the protests and hearings and recriminations that preceded the issuing of the Baby Doe regulations—"one might imagine that physicians and hospital administrators would be summarily executed if they violated the rule." And yet the regulations threaten neither criminal sanctions nor civil action. The penalty for breaking the new Baby Doe rules is... loss of federal child-abuse money. The incongruity between sin and sentence is at once astonishing and sensible. It seems the most reasonable way for politics to deal with so tortuous a moral issue: a strict standard and light punishment.

At the rawest cutting edge of moral life, the function of law should be not to punish, but to educate.

The rule, the suit, the debate, the fuss make me perversely optimistic. It is commonplace to claim that as our society has become more technologically advanced, we have become less and less sensitive to the value of human life: the technological imperative—an imperative for cleanliness, physical perfection, and ease—has made us insensitive to those human beings who don't fit the mold. Conservatives argue that society is conveniently disposing of those infirm at either end of life whose continued existence is a burden on society. I think not, or at least not more so than in other times. In previous ages, infant mortality was so high that it bred a certain callousness about the value of early life. Historian Joseph Kett writes: "Parents left their infants alone for long periods, seem to have been indifferent to their welfare, could not even remember their names, refused to attend the funerals of children under five, routinely farmed infants out for wet nursing, and argued in divorce proceedings, not over which parent could have the infant, but over which could send it packing." As for the severely deformed newborns, these were known as "monsters," and since "monsters were not [considered] human," says Kett, "their destruction was not viewed as murder." This is not just ancient history. It is reported that in England the rate of stillbirth of babies with spina bifida was 40 percent in 1958 and zero percent in 1962. It was between those two dates that treatment of the condition became possible. The stillbirths were almost certainly not stillbirths. They were obstetric euthanasia.

In fact, ours is a society enormously attentive to those in the dawn, the twilight, and the shadow of life, as Hubert Humphrey used to describe the young, the old, and the sick. And it is becoming increasingly attentive to the disabled newborn, who is all three. The Oklahoma doctors are learning that right now.

Part II Commentary

The Diversity of Theories of Moral Obligation and the Implications for Health Care Management

The abortion and neonatal cases make it clear that people have different views of moral goodness and that they feel very strongly about these. Obviously each position in these cases is compelling to those who hold it; the other views are clearly wrong. Yet all too painfully, all the groups feel exactly the same way. The differences that divide the case participants go to the foundations of moral thought. They demonstrate that although Americans share many concepts of what constitutes morality, they also have a number of serious differences.

Managers, who must get along with the widest possible spectrum of people to be effective, have a special reason to understand the nature of moral beliefs. The hospital organization and the manager's job require that all the participants live in the same organization or community. The manager of the abortion case hospital, like all managers, has a commitment to maintaining the health care of all the people in XYZ, despite their ethical differences. The secular not-for-profit tradition also calls for tolerating diversity of views, and making the hospital morally attractive to as many people as possible.

It is clear that these commitments will not be easy to honor. The depth of individuals' feelings precludes many of the devices we rely upon to resolve disputes. One side will not convince the other; open discussion on either the abortion or neonatal questions is more likely to strain relationships than produce agreement. A vote on the question will offend both parties and antagonize the losers. An appeal for funds to implement the donors' views will be inflammatory.

The Baby Doe question is closely related. The issue becomes one of accommodating views without damaging the rights or commitment of those who hold them. One way to explore the basic moral questions that these cases expose is to identify what are called theories of moral obligation. This commentary addresses what theories of moral obligation are, how they are used in organizational life, and how to deal with the conflict differing theories can create in health care organizations.

What Theories of Moral Obligation Are and How They Differ

One concept of ethics is based on the notion of duties or obligations that individuals hold. Kant's admonition is a statement of a duty, and many actors in the abortion and Baby Doe cases are pursuing what they perceive to be their duties. The concept of an ethics of duty drives the first three parts of this book, striving to identify the duties of the health care manager.

There are a great many theories of moral obligation, and philosophers have developed a complicated taxonomy to classify them. The first three categories are the *types* of theories of moral obligation, act versus rule *applications*, and the *origins* of moral obligation. To understand these, it is necessary also to review the *nature* of theories of moral obligation. Recognizing these distinctions is useful in devising a response to situations like the abortion case. Although the subject is of universal importance and formidable complexity, we will limit our discussion to some elementary lessons useful to managers. There is much we will be forced to omit, and the interested reader is encouraged to pursue Frankena's *Ethics* or other sources listed in the Suggested Readings, page xxiii.

The nature of theories of moral obligation

Ethics itself studies three questions:

1. What is a right act?
2. What should I do in a given situation? (It is possible that what should be done by a specific individual in a specific situation is one of a series of several right acts.)
3. What is good, or what is virtuous? (Right acts are clearly good, but intention must also be considered, as for example when the individual is ignorant of the need to act.)

Theories of moral obligation attempt to answer the first and second questions. (Theories of moral virtue attempt to answer the third question; we will return to these in Part IV.) To understand the different theories of moral obligation, it is necessary to consider a prior question: Just what do we mean by *good* and *right*?

It is clear that goodness has several dimensions. Material objects, for example, are good in the senses of being useful, attractive, saleable, efficient, symbolic, etc. That is, they make some contribution to a better material world. This is sometimes called *nonmoral goodness*. When we say, "Chevrolets are good cars," or "She makes good jewelry," we are talking about nonmoral goodness. People and ideas can be thought of as having nonmoral goodness, but they also have moral goodness over and above this. For example, "Joe is a good worker," and "Capitalism is a good form of economic organization," are at least ostensibly statements about nonmoral goodness. But Joe and capitalism inescapably have kinds of goodness that Chevrolets and jewelry do not. Joe may be kind, brave, humane, religiously observant, friendly. Capitalism may be is a better basis for personal freedom. These are moral dimensions of goodness, that is, they contribute to some higher goal than the material world alone. Actions similarly are right materially when they promote material goodness and right morally when they promote moral goodness. There might be no such thing as an act without moral rightness (or a person without moral goodness), but it is often helpful to identify the material or nonmoral, dimension to contrast it with the moral dimension.

The types of theories of moral obligation

Theories of moral obligation are beliefs that are intended to foster moral goodness, that is, the obligation, when fulfilled, will add to the moral goodness in the world. To the extent that it is not fulfilled, evil, the absence of moral goodness, will increase.

We can use the distinction between moral and nonmoral goodness in understanding the positions of the abortion case actors and others who are impelled by their personal theory of moral obligation. Some of the participants are talking about abortion in terms of its nonmoral impact: "There are too many people in this world already." "We're talking about children who can't possibly provide for the babies they're having." This pattern of thinking, deciding ethical or moral questions on their nonmoral goodness, is characteristic of teleological theories of moral obligation. The word *teleological* comes from the Greek *teleos*, meaning *end*. So teleological theories of obligation emphasize the result of the action. Most teleological theories evaluate the results in terms of a better material world. These are called *utilitarian* theories.

Other people arguing about abortion are not at all concerned with the material result, nonmoral goodness. For example, those who say "Abortion is killing, and 'Thou shalt not kill,' " or "A woman has an absolute right to her body," assume there is a compelling moral goodness that decides the issue. Whether killing will make a better society (like, for example, in a war against tyrants or the execution of murderers) is irrelevant, because "Thou shalt not kill." Similarly, for a different group, it does not matter whether the woman could raise a healthy child in a prosperous material setting: "A woman has an absolute right to her body." There is a characteristic to the logic that the goodness is self-evident; it is good because it is good. These are deontological theories of obligation. The word *deontological* comes from *deon*, the Greek word for "that which is binding."

Act versus rule applications

There is a second dimension to theories of moral obligation. They may apply to individual acts, such as the physician's "I have the right to decide who gets an abortion," which clearly suggests that case-by-case answers will be reached. Or they may apply universally, or nearly so, such as "Thou shalt not kill." Theories that apply to individual actions are called *act theories*. Those that attempt to be universal are called *rule theories*. To summarize, the first two dimensions of the taxonomy generate four major types of theories of moral obligation: act teleological, rule teleological, act deontological, and rule deontological.

The origins of theories of moral obligation

Note that *deontological* does not come from *deus*, the Latin for god, although the concept clearly bears some relation. Many deontological theories of moral obligation are based in religious belief; clearly one way to find out what is good because it is good is to seek God's advice. The person who said women have an absolute right to their bodies might have done that, or he or she might have developed the opinion from some other source. There are in fact three sources of theories of obligation: divine (God told me so, it says in God's testament, or it is in the dogma of my religion), personal (I simply believe it is so), and utilitarian (it promotes nonmoral goodness, the world will be a better place). Most theories or applications of theories contain clues about the origin. Utilitarians are revealed by their arguments. Instead of saying, "God tells us," or "I believe," they attempt to show that the world will be a better place. People pursuing morality based on religious beliefs frequently identify the divine origin. Without these clues, it is difficult to distinguish the origins of deontological beliefs. People following divine or personal insights can only be distinguished if they say so.

Obviously, there is great diversity in both personally inspired and divinely inspired moral theories. Personal theories encompass the extremes of racial hatred as well as Kant's maxim. Religious theories range from commitments to eliminate nonbelievers (religious wars, inquisitions, witch hunts) to the most inspiring examples of charity toward one's fellows (Gandhi, Albert Schweitzer, Mother Teresa). Both are familiar in major and long-established theologies.

Application of Theories of Moral Obligation

Although each individual has his or her own theory of moral obligation, it is often possible to understand where people are coming from when they state moral obligations. They use either teleological or deontological theories; they speak either to acts or as rules; and they derive their beliefs either from divine, personal, or utilitarian sources. While we differ in our ability to live up to these codes, it also appears that most people's theories are derived from a mixture of sources and are sometimes incomplete or contradictory. It is an interesting exercise to analyze the arguments in the abortion case. Hardly anyone sticks to a single, pure theory. Some people even say things that sound suspiciously contradictory, drawing willy-nilly on arguments that appear to support their position. You can also examine your own beliefs in terms of this taxonomy, gaining insights into why you hold certain feelings, and understanding how consistent and universal your positions are.

While individuals have great freedom, including the freedom to indulge in sloppy thought, organizations have greater responsibility. Their managers and leaders must accept more rigorous limits. Many practical situations require more than one theory to resolve. Act theories tend to be either too simplistic for some questions or too complicated to be practical. Rule theories often do not cover the specific case. This problem can be solved if one can extend the rules to make a consistent decision on the specific act, but that is not always easy. More seriously, it turns out that there are identifiable limitations in both teleological and deontological rule theories. Certain issues are too mundane to be included in many bodies of religious thought, such as whether you are obligated to educate your children. Others seem not to have been revealed, such as how to deal with organ transplants and persistent vegetative states. Similarly, utilitarian theories founder on questions of individual rights: is the greatest good for all worth the sacrifice of others? Slavery, colonialism, the sterilization of unfit persons, the use of fetal tissue for others, and capital punishment are all questions for which the greatest material good for society is not necessarily the greatest good for each member. The question whether society or the individual shall prevail is one of the vexing issues of life. Kant's maxim provides one answer; the individual is never to be used as a means to the end of social benefit. Other deontological theories are also helpful, such as Christ's principle, ". . . [A]s you did it to one of the least of my brethren, you did it to Me."[4] The point is that one must leave the context of teleological theory to resolve the question.

Some of the possible types and origins of theories are much more useful than others. It is hard even to think of a sensible example for *utilitarian deontology*; the words are contradictory. So is *divine teleology*. Some possibilities have not been popular, while others are cornerstones of most of our ethical thought. For example, *divine act deontology* requires that we await God's advice on each decision. It is followed by devout people who pray for wisdom on important events in their lives. *Personal act deontology*, meditating until some answer occurs to us (without weighing the nonmoral goodness of the results, which would change the theory to *personal act teleology*), has far fewer disciples.

Two types of theories recur throughout American and recent Western thought on public or community morality. They govern much of the behavior of organizations, both by law and by tradition. *Divine rule deontology* establishes many aspects of our daily lives, even for those who are not devout or observant. Much of common law is the application or extension of Judeo-Christian rules. So is a large part of our charitable activity. The rules establishing personal freedom in the Bill of Rights and the sometimes elaborate courtesies and compromises we make to live with the resulting differences are apparently deontological, with both personal and religious support (as in "Do unto others as you would have them do unto you," and Kant's maxim). *Rule utilitarian teleology* supports much of the rest of the U.S. Constitution and legislated law. The writings of James Madison and John Stuart Mill, who advanced many of the basic ideas of our government, clearly emphasize the advancement of nonmoral goodness as a goal. In many cases, both theories lead to the same conclusions. For example, truth telling is a deontological virtue, but it is also a foundation of economic enterprise.

Problems arise for society when two individuals pursue theories that conflict. The answer adopted by most Western nations is that one may pursue one's own beliefs as long as, and only as long as, they do not interfere with someone else's. Simply put, your rights stop at the end of my nose. The religious freedom guaranteed in the U.S. Bill of Rights is extended to moral freedom, but only as long as its exercise does not interfere with the rights of others. This approach is advocated as both a teleological (necessary to attain the material benefits of modern society) and deontological (simply the right way to live) rule. Most of us adopt this legal principle as a moral one; we tolerate religious and moral differences socially as well as legally. This tolerance is extended in our organizations. As part of the price of having the institutions, we tolerate compromise with the opinions of others that we might not accept in closer quarters, such as in our family.

Our tolerance is often strained. The compromises are painfully achieved, but we abide by them because the cost of social disruption would be worse. We have examples of the cost of other solutions available to us, such as those societies where religious conformity is central to all moral thought or where the ruling class, race, or party enforces its views on the rest of the society. The abortion case and the damaged neonates case are painful because they threaten the organizations involved with conflicts too serious to tolerate and too difficult to compromise. Under the pain of these conflicts, we sometimes abandon the material benefits of our institutions, and in the worst cases, we escape all introspective examination of these questions and simply act on an emotional basis. Violence is the most threatening of these emotional responses.

These problems give managers an extra burden. Managers accept society's commitment to moral consensus and a utilitarian obligation to support its organizations for their professional lives. Fortunately, these obligations rarely conflict with personal theories, but when they do, the conflict is painful. It is unlikely that managers, or other leaders such as trustees, can hold personal theories of moral obligation that radically depart from the prevailing views in our society. There are clearly limits to the amount of moral diversity that either an individual or an institution can tolerate.

Dealing with Conflict in Theories of Moral Obligation

Understanding the taxonomy of theories of obligation and the distinction between moral and nonmoral acts and ideas is useful for managers and anyone else who aspires to improve the world in either a material or a moral sense. The ability to tolerate moral diversity that grows from understanding might itself be a moral virtue, and it certainly is a nonmoral one that is valuable to health care managers.

Consequences of unresolved conflict

Can a hospital manager do nothing in the face of severe moral conflict? No, for two reasons. The first is that if the manager does nothing, the forces are liable to polarize further, dividing the board, the staff, the employees, and eventually the entire community. There is a real danger that the hospital will be impaired, or even destroyed, by this division. The forces engendered by different theories of moral obligation are historically violently destructive. The French and U.S. revolutions, the U.S. Civil War, and the Inquisition serve as examples; there are thousands throughout history, down to the repression of demonstrators in Tiananmen Square, Beijing, in 1989.

The second reason the manager in the abortion case must act is that she has a serious, unresolved ethical conflict of her own. Personal ethical conflict for managers is not uncommon. It is not clear scientifically what unresolved moral conflict will do to an individual, but there is nothing to suggest it does good. In literature, drama, history, and folk wisdom, there is the strong suggestion that ignoring one's moral beliefs is the foundation of tragedy, through retribution of the gods, bad luck, or the collapse of personality and health.

Some actions to avoid

Understanding the nature of moral conflict might not suggest what to do, but it often suggests some things to avoid. If we value the hospital as a moral institution in its own right, some actions are potentially destructive. Are we to educate people in the "right" way to think about abortion, damaged neonates, and similar moral problems? A nonreligious, not-for-profit hospital can educate people only to the extent that they consent; a governmental one must be even more circumspect. The best approaches are those that do not threaten moral beliefs directly, such as a review of the problem of supporting damaged and unwanted children. The organization may choose to avoid or defer some issues, proceeding at a conservative pace to minimize the potential danger to the institution. A town meeting, where some of the more committed believers might end up in a pitched battle with others, looks counterproductive. Is the hospital in the abortion case to hold a vote or survey over the right answer? No, because either outcome simply overrules the beliefs of the minority, without resolving them. To follow such a process and adopt the result would be to create a tyranny of the majority, either against the women seeking abortions or against those morally opposed to participating or tolerating them. Is the answer to ask the trustees to vote on the question? Not if it can be avoided. The action has the same weaknesses as a public vote and also smacks of a moral aristocracy. More practically, it could create stress among the board members that could impair the board for several years. None of these actions is promising; in one way or another, each threatens the moral rights of individuals, and several threaten the strength of the hospital.

Options for the health care executive

Some aspects of the administrator's predicament should now be clear. For one thing, it is far more severe than the usual nonmoral argument. People and institutions are sometimes damaged by nonmoral arguments and errors; they are rarely destroyed by them. If the abortion case were about whether to start a nursing home, and the neonate case were about whether to have a birthing center, the consequences might be severe, but the hospital and the administrator are likely to survive. In addition, talking about it, the usual way to resolve nonmoral disagreements, probably is dangerous here.

What can the poor executive do, then? It turns out that there are still three avenues open.

Avoidance. The best policy for a manager is clearly to avoid moral controversy whenever possible. It is often difficult to see how moral controversy might be avoided, but there are ways. The hospital may still announce that it will not make a decision. The effect is (1) to remove the question from the agenda and (2) to provide no service but also not to deny the women's rights. The moral argument in support of the position is that because the hospital itself represents an agreement to seek the common ground of moral consensus, it should not adopt a moral position that exceeds the consensus. The agreement itself and its extension to avoiding the abortion question arise from teleological grounds, but the agreement has already been explicitly or implicitly accepted by all the participants.

Separation. Separation strategies are a second possibility. These strategies simply follow an ancient axiom that it is better to part than to fight. Geographic or other forms of distance help. Perhaps the nurse who does not want to participate in abortions would be comfortable in the delivery room if the abortions were done in the outpatient clinic. The inevitable question is, How far is far enough? Many people seem to be able to live with solutions if they are not frequently confronted with what they believe to be abominations.

It is not always easy to see the separation possibilities, but they can be imagined. For example, the women's rights organization could provide transportation to the nearest city offering abortion. If the community is large enough, a free-standing abortion facility might be established by someone else. The doctor who feels so strongly about the question could be encouraged to perform first trimester abortions in his or her office. The pro-life supporters who cannot live with these actions of others must move in directions not involving the hospital. The pro-choice supporters must risk losing a partial victory if they press for a total one. If one of these solutions can be found, the board can be advised that the question is no longer important for the hospital.

Redefinition. It is occasionally possible to achieve a solution by sharpening the distinctions that define areas where agreement is possible. In abortion debates, extenuating circumstances (rape, incest, threatened life of the mother) have been tried as a redefinition with some success, but they apply only to a tiny fraction of the relevant cases. Other efforts to define life at later stages of fetal development, such as the twenty-first week (the youngest age for survival outside the uterus) or at quickening (when the fetus moves), have not been acceptable to all parties. Some other definitional possibilities include identifying abortion as a specific surgical procedure, excluding suction methods sometimes called menstrual regulation and abortifacient drugs. None of these proposals has satisfied the most committed antiabortion activists, but it is also clear that the size of the dissenting group is affected by the specific definitions.

Although redefinition has been of limited value in the abortion question, it was more useful in the damaged neonate question; identifying the expected specific types of treatment and specifying three criteria where heroic intervention would be inappropriate allowed a larger group of people to accept Baby Doe II. In the case of severely injured adults, the definition of *brain death* has permitted agreement on transplantation. Brain death is a refinement of the definition of death that is valuable precisely because it is acceptable to a broad consensus.

Other compromise. Avoidance, separation, and redefinition are forms of compromise that can be applied separately or together to resolve or ameliorate moral disagreements. The severely damaged neonates case illustrates the kind of opportunity that exists. The federal regulation still mandates that the hospital take a vigorous stance in defense of the neonate's life, independent of considerations of the quality of that life. However, the requirement for public display has been eliminated and the standards of proof required for violations have been raised. The largest compromise occurs in the penalty to the institution. Enforcement is changed from an action under civil rights law to withholding federal funds that, for child abuse, are insufficient anyway. The solution is logically and morally tortuous, and it is probably unsatisfactory to everyone who held an opinion in the original dispute. But it has removed the issue from the public agenda and avoided governmental intervention in many specific decisions.

Notes to Part II

1. Department of Health and Human Services, Child Abuse and Neglect Prevention and Treatment Program, 45 CFR Part 1340 (1985).
2. C. Krauthammer. "What To Do About Baby Doe," *The New Republic*, 2 September 1985, 20.
3. L. M. Kopelman, T. G. Irons, and A. E. Kopelman, "Neonatologists Judge the 'Baby Doe' Regulations" *New England Journal of Medicine* 318 (1988): 677–83.
4. Matthew 24:40.

Part III

Conflicting *Prima Facie* Obligations

Case 3

Providing References

Introductory Note: This relatively simple case is designed to show what conflicting moral obligations are and how quickly they can arise in management. In each situation, one can begin the analysis by identifying who might be used as a means, in Kant's sense, by various kinds of responses to the situations outlined. A little thought will show that obligations lie in several directions and that there is not likely to be a perfect solution. How then does the manager decide which solution is best? And how did the doctors from Harvard reach a decision that their peers felt compelled to censure?

There are several ethical considerations in the handling of information about other people. Each of the following situations has been constructed so that it might present an ethical dilemma to some. Please identify the major alternative views and the values that might be used to justify them. Then indicate how you would act.

1. A clerical employee under your direct supervision moves to another city. You get a telephone call for a reference. You know the good points—pleasant, usually reliable, thorough—and the bad—not too bright, relatively high absenteeism. How much do you reveal?

2. A written reference request is received regarding a nurse. You recently terminated the nurse because, although her work was adequate, repeated narcotic shortages arose on her shift. How much do you reveal?

54   Conflicting Prima Facie Obligations

3. The following article is reproduced in full from *The New York Times*, February 4, 1982.

3 Doctors Censured on Letters of Recommendation*

Boston, Feb. 3—The Massachusetts Medical Society said today that it had censured three doctors who wrote highly favorable letters of recommendation for a colleague recently convicted of raping a nurse. They were also placed on a year's probation.

In a related development, a Harvard Medical School committee released a report concluding that staff members had an obligation to report information about the "personal character" of physicians when recommending them for medical positions.

The report apparently marks the first time that prominent members of a major medical institution have explicitly stated that physicians have a responsibility to evaluate their colleagues' personal qualifications rather than simply their technical proficiency.

Dr. Stanley Wyman, president of the Massachusetts Medical Society, said that the censure and one-year probation had been imposed for the doctors' failure "to expose a fellow physician's deficiency in character."

'Continuing under supervision'

"It is simply a reprimand," Dr. Wyman added. "We want them to know that we are continuing them under supervision."

The physicians censured by the society's Ethics and Discipline Committee are Dr. Benjamin Covino, a professor at Harvard Medical School and chief anesthesiologist at Brigham and Women's Hospital; Dr. Aaron Gissen, also an anesthesiologist at the hospital, and Dr. John Wark, who left the hospital last year and now practices in Nevada.

All three wrote letters of recommendation in behalf of Dr. Arif Hussain, a former resident at Brigham and Women's, who used the

---

The New York Times, 4 February 1982, sec. IV, p. 27. Copyright © 1982 by The New York Times Company. Reprinted by permission.

letters to gain an appointment at Children's Hospital in Buffalo. The letters made no mention of the fact that Dr. Hussain was one of three physicians convicted last year in a Boston rape case.

The incident touched off a dispute between the Buffalo hospital, which revoked Dr. Hussain's appointment, and the Boston hospitals.

The Massachusetts Medical Society does not have the power to revoke a physician's license. But Dr. Wyman said that because the doctors wrote the letters partly at the advice of the legal counsel at Brigham and Women's, their action "was nothing that remotely warrants" revocation of their licenses by the state's Board of Registration in Medicine.

Dr. Hussain and his two co-defendants in the rape case were sentenced to three to five years in Walpole State Prison, but the sentences were suspended. Since his conviction, Dr. Hussain has been charged in another Boston rape case, occurring in 1978 and involving patients.

The controversy over the letters written for Dr. Hussain prompted Daniel C. Posteson, the dean of Harvard Medical School, to appoint a 14-member committee to suggest guidelines for the preparation of letters of recommendation. The committee's report, written Jan. 11 but not released by the school until today, makes five specific recommendations that must be approved by the school's faculty.

Its primary suggestion is that physicians follow a "golden rule" of letter writing. "This means," it says, "that a letter should contain the information known to the writer which he would like to have were he to receive the letter."

Such information should include anything bearing on the doctor's ability to perform his duties, the report said. "Information regarding personal character is of great importance in the case of physicians," it continued, "and particularly for physician teachers."

In recent years, doctors have become increasingly wary of what they say in such letters, for fear that critical comments could result in costly lawsuits.

Addressing those fears, the Harvard committee's report noted that if the letters "contain factual information and opinion that has been arrived at in a careful and reasonable fashion, such suits will be very unlikely to prevail."

Case 4

The Doctor, the Patient, and the DRG

Introductory Note: One of the most common points of conflict between *prima facie* obligations is that arising from the duty to one patient versus the duty to all patients. It arises here in financial form: When is it appropriate to curtail access to resources (in this case, vaginal delivery) for some patients (in this case, the patients of one doctor) to ensure access to all services for all patients, present and future? In addition to the questions posed at the end of the case, consider how the DRG management problem can be handled to minimize this kind of moral conflict.

The Doctor, the Patient, and the DRG*

by Jeffrey Wasserman

Lakeview Hospital in central New Jersey has been reimbursed on the basis of "diagnosis related groups," or DRGs... since May 1980. The hospital's medical director, Jared Lapin, M.D., acts as a liaison between the hospital's managers and the medical staff. In

---

*Reprinted from *The Hastings Center Report*, October 1983, p. 23. Reproduced by permission. © The Hastings Center.

addition, Dr. Lapin and Ellen O'Connor, director of finance, periodically review the performance of individual physicians from a financial viewpoint.

At a recent meeting, Dr. Lapin and Ms. O'Connor analyzed a lengthy computer report that matched, for each physician, the revenue the hospital received with the costs incurred for treating patients in each of the DRGs in one month. While studying the fifteen DRGs under Major Diagnostic Category number 14 (Pregnancy, Childbirth, and the Puerperium), they noticed that Dr. Daniel Weiner admitted seventeen patients who were later determined to be in DRG 373 (vaginal delivery without complicating diagnosis) but only two in DRG 371 (cesarian section, without complication and/or comorbidity). Yet for the other three obstetricians on staff, fifty-eight came under DRG 373 and nineteen under 371. Across all deliveries, the costs of treating Dr. Weiner's patients exceeded the revenue received from the DRG rates. But the total cost incurred in providing care to the other obstetricians' patients was considerably below revenue and hence the hospital was able to earn a "profit."

The computer report also revealed that the reimbursement rate the hospital received for routine deliveries fell just short of covering all the incurred expenses, whereas the rate paid for cesarian sections was substantially greater than the actual cost to the hospital. The reason for Dr. Weiner's comparatively poor overall "financial performance," Dr. Lapin and Ms. O'Connor concluded, was that he performed many fewer cesarians than did his colleagues.

Dr. Weiner explained that he did not agree with his colleagues that once a woman had a cesarian delivery, all subsequent deliveries must be cesarian; he felt that most of these women could have normal deliveries. He cited a number of recent studies that found no differences in outcomes (in terms of health risks to both mother and child) associated with the different delivery modes. Dr. Lapin countered that the tradition of performing repeat cesarians was strong and that more time and research were needed before large numbers of physicians changed their practices. He noted too that, if a complication were to arise, the attending physician would likely be faced with a malpractice suit.

Finally, he pointed out to Dr. Weiner that the hospital was losing money on almost every patient he treated. "Dan," he said, "its in all our interests to look out for the financial health of the hospital. And since it is unclear which of the two approaches benefits the patient more, I urge you to reconsider the way you handle these cases."

Was it ethical for Dr. Lapin to approach Dr. Weiner if there was no indication he was delivering poor quality care? How should financial considerations, both those related to the hospital and society at large, be weighed against physician judgment? What if Dr. Weiner could convincingly demonstrate that his patients were actually at less risk than those of his colleagues?

Case 5

Terminating the Employment Contract—The Abortion Case, Part Two

Introductory Note: Organizations are a form of moral consensus, and conflicts can occur when the individual's views depart from the consensus. This case illustrates two important forms. First, what are the rights of staff to hold values toward abortion and the obligations of the organization to respond? What can or should be done for the nurse, especially if the hospital opts to provide abortions directly? The law apparently holds that he or she may be discharged, but is this the wisest action?

Second, when do moral concerns justify terminating an executive's relationship to the institution? Who should terminate it, and on what terms? Are there conditions when an executive may not terminate the relationship, even though he or she wishes to?

You personally have the conviction that abortion is wrong, although you have never attempted to analyze the source of your feelings or to influence the national political argument. As you sort through the arguments, you realize that you might affect the outcome even by the content and structure of your report. On the

---

This case was prepared by Peter A. Wilson, Ph.D., and John R. Griffith.

one hand you can honor your personal belief and make a strong case against the feasibility of the project that you feel you can sell to the volunteers, thereby quashing the project. On the other hand, is it proper to impose your values on the organization?

Not only would you like to resolve this particular dilemma but you wonder about the whole question of the proper relation between your professional obligation as custodian of the organization and your obligations and values as a person and citizen.

Is it reasonable to remain with the organization if abortion is permitted? On the other hand, what is your obligation to the organization where, until a few days ago, you were quite happy? May you simply walk out? Are there terms on which you can stay, or terms under which you are obligated to stay?

The next day when you arrive at work (at the hospital described in Case 1), one of the obstetric nursing supervisors is in your waiting room. She feels that abortion is a great evil and that she can have nothing to do with it. Even the discussion has been very upsetting, and she would like to be transferred. With a few calls you ascertain that there are no appropriate vacancies for her. The County Nurses' Association says that it is not right to penalize the nurse for her beliefs. The County Nurses' Association has no collective bargaining contract with your hospital, but it has been an aggressive advocate of nurses' rights and would like certification as a union.

Case 6

The End of Life: Assisting Families and Clinical Personnel with Terminal Care

Introductory Note: Doctors and nurses daily face the dilemma that is graphically described in the following case. When life is clearly coming to an end, what is the best role for our complicated, expensive health care system? One strict deontological position is that "everything possible" must always be done for the individual patient under your care, but this position ignores three issues others think important. First, the patient might not want everything or, if no longer competent, like the patient in the case, might not have wanted it if he or she had the capacity to judge. Second are the larger ramifications of doing everything. Where will the resources come from? Some argue they come from the poor and uninsured, that if we reduced the amount we spend on those who are dying, roughly 15 percent of all hospital expenses, we would have more for those without access to care. And finally, do we have any obligations to the family members, for their time, funds, or pain and suffering?

Managers must recognize the reality of the dilemma and look beyond it to another issue. No matter what your belief about managing the end of life, the staff who face these issues at the bedside are entitled to understanding support. What can management do for Dr. Hilfiker and Ginger?

Facing Our Ethical Choices*

by David Hilfiker, M.D.

The phone wakes me; it is 3 a.m.

"Hello, Dr. Hilfiker? This is Ginger at the nursing home. Mrs. Toivonen has a fever."

Despite my tiredness my mind is immediately clear. Elsa Toivonen, 83 years old. Confined to the nursing home ever since her stroke three years ago. Bedridden. Aphasic. In an instant I remember her as she was before the stroke: her dislike and distrust of doctors and hospitals, her staunch pride and independence despite her severe scoliosis, her wry grin every time I suggested hospitalization for some problem. I remember admitting her to the hospital after her stroke, one side completely paralyzed, globally aphasic, incontinent, and reduced to helplessness. And I remember those first few hospital days in which I aggressively treated the pneumonia that developed as a complication, giving her intravenous antibiotics despite her apparent desire to die. "Depressed," I had thought. "She'll get over it. Besides, she may recover substantially in the next few weeks." She recovered from the pneumonia, but she remained paralyzed and aphasic. For the past three years she had lain curled in her nursing-home bed, a grim reminder of the "power" of modern medicine.

"David?" Ginger's voice brings me back to my tired body.

"Oh... yes. Any other symptoms?" I know already that I'm going to have to go in, but I try to postpone the decision for a few minutes.

"Well, it's hard to tell. She hasn't been eating much the last few days, and she's had a little cough. Her temp started during the evening."

"What's her temperature now?"

"One hundred three point five, rectally."

"Oh... all right," I say reluctantly. "I'll be right in."

Ginger is waiting for me in the dark hall of the nursing home,

---

*Excerpted from D. Hilfiker, "Allowing the Debilitated to Die: Facing Our Ethical Choices," *New England Journal of Medicine* 308 (1983): 716–17. Reprinted with permission, *New England Journal of Medicine.*

just outside Mrs. Toivonen's room, chart in hand. "She looks pretty sick, David."

She does, indeed! Wasted away to 69 lb., decubitus ulcers on her back and hip, peering at me from behind her blank face—I'm used to all that from my monthly rounds. But this morning there is no movement of her eyes, no resistance to my examination, nothing to indicate that she is really there. There is little more to the history of Mrs. Toivonen's fever than what I gathered over the phone, and her aphasia precludes much of an interview. My examination is brief, directed pointedly toward the usual causes of fever in the elderly. (I remember the *Journal* article* suggesting that nursing-home patients received less thorough attention simply because they were debilitated. It's true, of course, and I can't defend it, but I know that if Joe Blow, 47-year-old schoolteacher, were in the emergency room with a fever I would be spending an hour talking with him and examining him thoroughly.) I try to assuage my guilt with the thought that I can't exhaust myself now in the middle of the night if I'm going to be able to give decent care to all the other patients, beginning at eight in the morning.

Listening to Mrs. Toivonen's chest, I hear the expected rales, and I complete the rest of the examination without finding anything else.

"I think she's got pneumonia," I say to Ginger, and we both look down at Mrs. Toivonen's withered body. I wonder to myself what I'm going to do now.

I ask Ginger to call the technician out of bed for a chest x-ray, and I write orders for a urine culture. While waiting for the x-ray, Ginger and I sit at the nurses' station, writing our respective reports.

Ginger looks up. "Mabel Lundberg said she hoped there wouldn't be any heroics if Mrs. Toivonen got sick again."

"I know," I answer. "She talked with me. What does she mean by 'heroics'?" Mabel is the only friend Mrs. Toivonen has, her only visitor; she probably knows better than anyone what Mrs. Toivonen would really want. But the only relative, a distant niece living in another state, has called some months ago asking that "everything possible" be done for her aunt. "Everything possible," "heroics": it all depends on the words you choose.

Essentially alone, foggy from tiredness in the middle of the night, I will make decisions that will probably mean life or death for this poor

---

*Brown NK, Thompson DJ. Nontreatment of fever in extended-care facilities. N Engl J Med. 1979;300:1246–50.

old woman. I think back to medical school and university hospital, where $1,000 worth of laboratory and x-ray studies would have been done to make sure she really did have pneumonia: several views of the chest, urine cultures, blood cultures, throat cultures, sputum for stain and culture (obtained by inducing this 69-lb, 83-year-old lady to expectorate or by transtracheal aspiration), blood counts, Mantoux test, lung scans to rule out emboli—the list is only as limited as one's imagination. And each study is "reasonable" if we really mean to be thorough; I can almost hear the residents suggesting obscure possibilities to demonstrate their erudition. (And they are not wrong, either. Can any price be put on a human life? Is it not worth anything to discover a rare, potentially fatal, but curable illness?)

There in the middle of the night I consider "doing everything possible" for Mrs. Toivonen: transfer to the hospital, intravenous lines for hydration and antibiotics, thorough laboratory and x-ray evaluation, twice-daily rounds to be sure she is recovering, more toxic antibiotics, and even transfer to our regional hospital for evaluation and care by a specialist. None of it is unreasonable, and another night I might choose just such a course. But tonight my human sympathies lie with Mrs. Toivonen and what I perceive as her desire to die. Perhaps it's because Ginger is working, and I know how impatient she is with technologic heroics; perhaps it's because I've been feeling a little depressed myself in the past few days; perhaps, I think to myself, it's because I'm tired and lazy and don't want to bother. In any event I decide against the heroics.

But I can't just do nothing, either. My training and background are too strong. I do not allow myself to be consistent and just go home. Compromising (and ultimately making a decision that makes no medical or ethical sense at all), I write orders instructing the nursing staff to administer liquid penicillin, to encourage fluid intake, and to make an appointment with my office so I can reexamine Mrs. Toivonen in 36 hours. On my way out of the dark hospital, I talk with the x-ray technician and check the x-ray film: It is questionable at best. With her severe scoliosis Mrs. Toivonen is always difficult to x-ray, and the chronic changes in her lungs make early inflammation difficult to detect. I thank the technician for the x-ray, wondering to myself why I ordered it. Driving home, I wonder why practicing medicine is so often dissatisfying; as usual it takes me an hour to get back to sleep.

Case 7

Tough Transplant Questions Raised by Baby Jesse Case

Introductory Note: Whenever new medical technology emerges, it goes through a period of development when it can be available only to some potential recipients, raising the *prima facie* question, Which one? Transplants are a particularly complicated example of this problem. The supply will always be limited, and there are serious ethical questions involved in getting donor commitment and handling the logistics. (Note carefully the actions of Butterworth Hospital and the regional organ procurement agency.) Then comes the core issue: If you have a heart that is appropriate for either Baby Calvin or Baby Jesse, who decides, and on what criteria?

Tough Transplant Questions Raised by 'Baby Jesse' Case*

by Marcia Chambers

Los Angeles, June 14—It is the stuff of soap operas, but it raises difficult moral questions that affect the most helpless of patients: newborns. The issues all center on what factors determine who gets the few hearts available for transplant.

---

*The New York Times, 15 June 1986, sec. I, p. 16. Copyright © 1986 by The New York Times Company. Reprinted by permission.

The young, unwed parents beg Loma Linda University Medical Center to perform a heart transplant on their desperately ill son. The hospital turns them down, apparently because they are not married. Then it reconsiders, but only after the parents agree to sign over custody of their 3-week-old infant to his paternal grandparents. They fly to New York to make a public plea for a heart on the Phil Donahue talk show. Midway in the program last Tuesday, a telephone call comes from Butterworth Hospital in Grand Rapids, Mich.

Tears and applause

"We are donating a heart to the baby in Loma Linda, California," says Gera Witte, a spokesman for the hospital.

The audience bursts into tears and applause. The young parents, Jesse Sepulveda, 26, and Deana Binkley, just turned 17, embrace. Susan Carpenter McMillan, California spokesman for the National Right to Life Committee, who publicized the young couple's plight, shrieks. The Rev. Michael Carcerano, the parish priest who baptized Jesse, smiles.

Within minutes, the parents and their entourage are whisked off stage, and Mr. Donahue tells his audience that the hospital's announcement had not been arranged before the program. Soon the group is flying for California, to Loma Linda University Medical Center, the nation's leading experimental center for infant heart transplants, 60 miles south of Los Angeles.

Meanwhile, Baby Jesse, born May 25, is being transferred from Huntington Memorial Hospital in Pasadena to Loma Linda. And the brain-dead infant known as Baby Frank is being transferred by air from Butterworth Hospital in Grand Rapids to Loma Linda.

Apparently neither doctors at Loma Linda nor those at Butterworth knew that another baby, Robert Dean Cardin, initially known as Baby Calvin of Kentucky, was next on the national organ procurement list to receive a heart. The Kentucky baby had been bypassed, it turns out, because of a miscommunication between a Butterworth physician and a regional organ procurement agency in Michigan.

As a result, the heart surgeon for the Kentucky baby turned to news organizations, and the baby received a new heart Friday in Louisville.

The national organ system, which has evolved over the years as hospitals have sought ways to find donors for adults and, more recently, infants, has evoked criticism from a variety of quarters. Senator Albert

Gore Jr., of Tennessee, said: "What do we tell families such as these? That they have to go on the Phil Donahue show? Is this the best we can do?"

Some troubling issues

According to ethicists around the country, the drama has raised troubling questions in infant heart transplants, a field that is experimental. The questions include these:

- Should a hospital be permitted to use social factors to reject a child in need of a heart? Initially, Baby Jesse was rejected not for medical reasons but for social reasons. The social guidelines used by Loma Linda include the ability of the parents to understand and follow a complex treatment program after the transplant. The guidelines also bar those parents with a history of drug or alcohol abuse, or of mental illness.
- Have the communications media become a participant in the story of Baby Jesse and other babies? Is it true, as one social scientist said, that the family who commands the media, commands the heart?
- Was the national network system of donor procurement bypassed in this case, when the donor's parents designated their baby's heart for Jesse?
- How does a hospital arrive at a policy on what the public should be told that also takes into account the privacy of patients and their families? Citing confidentiality standards, Loma Linda was unable to rebut Right to Life statements that Baby Jesse was rejected as a transplant patient because of the couple's unwed status and the youth of the mother. The hospital finally denied the reasons put forth by Mrs. McMillan, and, while not specifying its reasons, spoke of the extraordinary role required of parents in the post-operative care of these infants.

'Awesome responsibility'

Underlying those issues is the reality that hearts for transplants, particularly infant hearts, are very scarce, prompting hospitals to be extremely selective.

"More than 100 people are involved in a transplant operation such as the one for Baby Jesse, and we can't waste that amount of time and resources if there is a chance the caretakers aren't up for an awesome responsibility," said Dr. Leonard Bailey, the Loma Linda surgeon who performed the transplant operation on Baby Jesse.

Dr. Bailey and others on the 20-member committee that reviews transplant candidates said the panel's initial decision against an operation for Baby Jesse, which members said was unanimous, had nothing to do with his parents' age or marital status. Dr. Bailey performed the first baboon-to-baby heart transplant at Loma Linda in 1984 on an infant known as Baby Fae, and in that case the parents were separated.

At a news conference Thursday, the surgeon noted that postoperative care was crucial to recovery. "It's not good enough to go off in a corner, take a Valium and hope it all goes away," he said, adding that the possibility that the transplanted heart will be rejected by the body is constant and requires aggressive parental attention. "The family has to be very dependable," he said.

While the hospital will not say why Jesse's parents were rejected, several members of the transplantation committee said privately that the mother had "substance abuse" problems. Miss Binkley, Jesse's mother, could not be reached for comment.

Social factors called valid

Arthur Caplan, associate director of the Hastings Center in New York, a research institute that studies ethical problems in health care, said he thought the use of psychosocial and familial factors was "extremely valid" in assessing candidates for transplant.

Baby Jesse, who was described today as "alert and active" and "progressive well" after his surgery Tuesday night, was born May 25 at Huntington Memorial Hospital in Pasadena with hypoplastic left heart syndrome, a congenital defect that is usually fatal. Neonatal specialists at Huntington turned immediately to Loma Linda, which has performed five infant heart transplants, more than any other facility in the country, since it began the program six months ago.

The parents were interviewed by a psychiatrist at Loma Linda, according to members of the transplantation committee. The mother's records, including information she gave to social workers, was examined. In a unanimous vote, the committee rejected the couple, members said.

Visit to their priest

Their parish priest, Mr. Carcerano in Pasadena, where the couple have lived for the last year, said the couple told him they heard about it from their physician at Huntington hospital. "The reason he gave was they were young and unwed," he said.

"I was disturbed by that reasoning," the priest said in an interview. After visiting the Huntington physician to confirm the account, "I then contacted the Right to Life group," he said.

He said the couple's decision to go public came in conversations with him and with Mrs. McMillan of the Right to Life group. On the Donahue program, Mrs. McMillan said in response to a question that she was called in "to alert the press" to Baby Jesse's story.

Dr. David Rothman, who oversees an ethics and science center at Columbia University's College of Physicians and Surgeons, said on the Donahue program and in an interview that he was outraged that psychosocial reasons had been used to initially deny Jesse a heart. "Generally, heart transplant teams lean over backwards to make sure that social criteria does not determine acceptability," Dr. Rothman said.

But Roger Evans, a medical sociologist at the Battelle Institute in Seattle, who is one of the nation's experts on heart and liver transplant issues, disagreed, saying social factors were relevant to the selection process.

"The concern is to make the best use of the heart," he said.

At the same time, Dr. Evans, as well as officials at organ transplant agencies around the country, were furious that an available heart was designated for a particular recipient, outside the normal organ procurement process. The national procurement process involves the matching of donors and recipients through use of computer lists and through record-keeping by regional agencies.

"Designating recipients is generally not considered an acceptable procedure," said Dr. Evans, a sentiment stated by others in almost the same words.

However, Dr. James Walters, an associate professor of Christian ethics at Loma Linda University, said: "Ultimately it is the parent who decides whether to donate or not to donate. If they choose not to donate, there is no heart. I think the parent who donates can say where it goes."

Miss Witte, the Butterworth Hospital spokesman, said in an interview that physicians at Butterworth had notified the regional organ procurement agency in Michigan.

She said the parents of Baby Frank, whose name was Frank Edward Clemenshaw, at first reluctant to agree to a heart donation, finally agreed to donate the heart to Jesse, after learning from television news reports that their son and Baby Jesse were born on the same day and that both couples were not married. Miss Witte said Baby Frank's parents had considered naming their child Jesse.

Last Monday, the day before Baby Jesse's parents appeared on the Donahue program, doctors at Butterworth notified doctors at Loma Linda about the donor heart available for Baby Jesse. "Loma Linda did not agree immediately to the donor," Miss Witte said. This was possibly because Dr. Bailey was out of the country that day.

And so the physician for the Baby Frank family telephoned the regional organ procurement agency in Michigan, according to Miss Witte. "The doctor mentioned he had already called Loma Linda," she said. She said this was apparently misunderstood and "the organ agency thought we had already made a commitment to Loma Linda."

"So they did not tell us" about the Kentucky baby, she went on. "It was a miscommunication."

Miss Witte said that because Loma Linda had the information about the donor on Monday, she thought the parents had been notified before they appeared on the Donahue program. In fact, according to Anita Rockwell, a Loma Linda spokesman, the hospital agreed to accept the Butterworth heart on Monday night but did not notify Baby Jesse's parents or grandparents until Tuesday morning.

Miss Witte said she received a telephone call from the Donahue producers, who told her that they had learned "we had a baby for Loma Linda" and that the parents were on the show.

She said that after some pressing from the producers, she agreed to say on the program that "we were donating a heart."

"The next thing I know Donahue is introducing me," Miss Witte said.

Part III Commentary

Dealing with Conflicting Moral Obligations—Negotiating the Slippery Slope

How Conflicting Obligations Arise

The cases for this chapter have three characteristics in common. First, they are representative of commonplace, almost daily events. The problems represented by these cases arise much more frequently than the conflicts between theories of moral obligation that underlie the abortion case and the newborn case. Second, with the exception of some of the end-of-life and transplant questions, the potential right acts are much less controversial. They tend to arise from theories of moral obligation that have broad, near-universal acceptance. Third, the real problems have no easy resolution. It is usually obvious that no matter how desirable the right acts might be, we cannot do them all. The painful part is not the theory; it is in deciding the specifics.

In this chapter we address the second of the three questions of ethics, What should I do? The initial list of obligations in problems like these, the right acts implied by moral theories, are called *prima facie* obligations. Obviously, if I can, I should fulfill *prima facie* obligations. But as the economists say about free lunches, and for many of the same reasons, there's no such thing as fulfilling them all. As a result, under the pursuit of Kant's rule, some individual is at risk to be used as a means to some other end. Thus the moral challenge shifts from identifying right acts to selecting among them.

Those who prefer absolute answers to moral questions call the weighing of conflicting *prima facie* obligations "the slippery slope," implying that properly humble mortals should not risk the moral consequences of error. "Where does it stop," they say. "If you judge this case and then the next, and the next, pretty soon you'll be doing something everybody would agree is unconscionable."

This chapter takes a different position. For the modern manager, there is no escape from the slippery slope. Dangerous as it is, the challenge is to negotiate it wisely. Conflicts among *prima facie* obligations are more common, and may be more complex, as a result of medicine's technological advances. Just a generation ago, cardiac surgery was experimental and the opportunity to transplant organs did not exist; terminal care was given by families at home; and without Medicare or Medicaid, over a third of all Americans were without financial access to health care. At least three of the five cases could not have existed. The slippery slope is a consequence of the advancing technology in health care and the economy in general.

The essay that follows develops three concepts for negotiating the slippery slope. First, these conflicts, like competition over scarce resources, are amenable to techniques of effective nonmoral management. Second, the cases are reviewed to show the applicability of accepted theories of management not only to resolving the conflicts themselves, but also to preventing or reducing similar conflicts. Third, a general guide is developed for dealing with *prima facie* conflicts. To do this requires some specific theory of moral obligation; the one chosen should be acceptable to most readers. Finally, there is a brief comment on the obligation to assume moral leadership in the face of opposition.

Relationship between *Prima Facie* Conflicts and Nonmoral Management

Conflicting *prima facie* obligations create painful dilemmas and the opportunity for great moral harm; the slope is truly slippery. But because they occur more often and can be easier to resolve than conflicts between theories of moral obligation, they offer a great opportunity for health care managers. While the abortion case might challenge the manager's skills in preventing the organization from destroying itself, these cases offer the challenge of doing better, of coming closer, more often, to the Kantian ideal.

Our first need, as managers, is to understand how central the moral problem of conflicting *prima facie* obligations is to the profession. It closely resembles the mundane problem of choosing among conflicting nonmoral opportunities for resource allocation. Selection is a central activity of management, politics, and economics, and moral selection is a different application rather than a new concept. That is to say, resolving *prima facie* obligations is an intrinsic part of what managers do for a living. Two important conclusions follow. First, these problems will be addressed with methods, processes, and technology similar to those used in most management activity. Second, it follows that bad management is inherently less moral than good management.

The nonmoral decision-making role of managers emphasizes processes to identify and select alternatives that yield the largest contribution to organizational goals while enhancing the participation and sense of reward of individual members.[1] The skills that contribute to this role include fact-finding; analysis; communication; the ability to accept new perspectives; and the flexibility to redefine, integrate, and imagine unexpected solutions. The better an individual or organization is at these skills, the higher the probability of finding the truly superior solution in either a moral or nonmoral context. And the better the process of search and dialogue is managed, the higher the nonmoral rewards of reaching the decision.

From this argument it follows that the first rule for resolving conflicting *prima facie* obligations is to run a good nonmoral organization. The stronger the organization is, the more resources it will acquire and the stronger its decision processes will be. A strong organization can satisfy a larger set of *prima facie* obligations because it has more resources and can tolerate more stress in examining conflicts because it is more skilled at conflict management. Thus a weaker organization is inherently less moral than a strong one. (Unfortunately, it does not follow that good management is inherently moral. The fascist Mussolini was famous for his management. He made the trains run on time, but he also persecuted Jews and dissidents like many other tyrants.)

How Good Nonmoral Management Contributes to Solving the Cases

The cases illustrate the tie between resolving the moral dilemmas and generally accepted practices of sound management.

Reference letters (Case 3)

Giving references is a commonplace activity, yet many people have difficulty with it, as the responses of the Harvard physicians indicate. As usual, the obligations are not hard to identify in the abstract. They lie to the individual being discussed, to the organization where the individual worked, to self, to the organization requesting information, and to society as a whole.

Truth-telling will go far to meet all these needs. To be fair and to protect against legal action, one will want not to either whitewash or malign the individual. Evidence that only the truth was told will discourage lawsuits and provide an absolute defense if they are brought. Rigorous truth-telling rules out communicating gossip or speculation and probably improves the overall quality of references.

But where does truth-telling interfere with privacy, and how does one judge the relative obligation to the inquirer and the individual? Most people would apply two universalization tests. They should tell any truth that they would feel relevant if the situation were reversed and they were the inquirer. Simultaneously, they should conceal any truth they would feel an invasion of their privacy if they were the individual. Where the two tests conflict, most people would use some calculus of the greatest good for the greatest number. Since many individuals could be exploited by concealing information that seriously threatens the quality of care—as a history of either rape or possible narcotics abuse would—the conclusion would be to release all factual information on these matters. (The factual information on the nurse is only that "repeated... shortages arose on her shift.")

Why is giving this information so difficult? There appears to be a human temptation to put more weight on the individual and less on the larger groups. The moral challenge for the manager is to discourage this tendency and in so doing both preserve the system of honest references and protect the individuals from embarrassment. A number of standard organizational devices can be used to meet this challenge. Procedures and guidelines can suggest the appropriate topics for references. Supervisory training can raise the issue with those likely to receive requests. A central office can provide counseling for referees, review the responses, or even process them, as undergraduate colleges assemble reference dossiers on graduates.

DRG management (Case 4)

The issue of DRG case management is the classic "guns versus butter" conflict of political economics, rewritten as "deficit versus health care." The case translates the problem to the microlevel, where patient care is delivered. The process by which New Jersey resolved the resource allocation question—that is, established DRGs—is one few of us wish to overthrow, and the problem becomes one of living morally within it.

The obligations lie to Dr. Weiner, his patients, other doctors, other patients, and the institution itself. Overall, the hospital must rationalize its obstetrics cost, but it must do this in ways that do not use any individual as a means to that end. It is important to note that the DRG pricing and length-of-stay decisions were not made in a moral vacuum. There is a serious misreading of the law and of the statistical reality inherent in assuming, as Dr. Lapin implicitly does, that the standard applies to any individual patient or doctor. The law and the regulations speak only to averages and specifically forbid harm to individuals. The statistical reality is the central limit theorem, which states that samples of sufficient size, drawn from the same underlying population, will have similar averages. Dr. Lapin has apparently not considered either whether Dr. Weiner's patients are sufficient in number to make judgments or are in fact drawn from the same population. (If for example, Dr. Weiner routinely refers all his questionable cases to other doctors on the staff, he will have a nonrepresentative sample with no Cesarian sections, but the hospital rate will not change.)

When the question is analyzed more carefully, the moral dilemmas originally posed disappear. The issue is not whether Dr. Weiner should do more Cesarians but whether the hospital can operate obstetrics effectively. In the case, no thought seems to have been given to the overall performance of the obstetrical group or the medical staff as a whole. It is quite likely that the doctors as a group can improve their cost-effectiveness using techniques like Deming's Total Quality Management.[2] If they can, there is no need to penalize Dr. Weiner and his patients. But what if the cost problem still persists after diligent efforts? One might appeal to the New Jersey system for a more equitable rate. Finally, one could consider either closing or expanding the obstetrics unit; larger units tend to be more economical because fixed costs are more widely spread.

That these actions—new behavior for all obstetricians, greater efficiency from hospital personnel, lobbying for a rate adjustment, or closing or expanding obstetrics service—are difficult is in fact the moral challenge of health care management. We are a profession because we are expected to be and are able to deal with such challenges.

The moral grounds for resignation and termination (Case 5)

In the abortion case, the obligations are to self, family, hospital, society, and, under the administrator's beliefs, to unborn children. The manager's need to resign must be weighed against her commitment to lead the organization, recognizing that well over 95 percent of the hospital's activities have nothing to do with abortion. If she is absolutely opposed to abortion in any situation, there is almost no conflict. The only question will be timing; she also has the obligation to remain working on other matters as long as other patients' welfare is at risk. Let us examine the conflict at its most serious, where the obligation to stay and the obligation to go are nearly balanced.

How does the nonmoral capability of the organization come into the question? If the decision is to resign, the impact on her career and the hospital will depend on relatively subtle aspects of the corporate culture, but well-managed institutions will do better. There will be subordinates trained to take over, a more attractive position for recruiting a successor, and outplacement to ease the transition. Second, in weighing the moral consequences of staying, the hospital that is a good place to work, is tolerant of individual viewpoints, and has been loyal to its workers in the past will tend to get the benefit of the doubt. Third, the better managed institution will be able to find and implement the innovative solution, say by turning the matter over to a deputy or a respected board member, and removing abortions and the debate to elsewhere in the community.

The obstetric supervisor's problem can be treated entirely on a nonmoral level, like a human resources management problem where the employee's health or home life make certain duties impossible. The obligations are to the supervisor, other employees, and the institution. Good organizations try to keep individuals who have made a contribution, because it is a form of reward that is often appreciated by many more than are directly involved. The ability to place the individuals successfully in appropriate other work will depend on the organization's relationship to its workers, its retraining programs, and flexibility in managing its work force. If no suitable placement can be found, the organization can assist with outplacement services.

Terminal care (Case 6)

The problems of terminal care raised so graphically by Dr. Hilfiker are common now and will become more so as our population ages. The principle obligations are to the patient and to society. (Although one might begin with a rule that the patient's needs must come first, the money spent on Ms. Toivonen comes from a meager supply that is essentially fixed in the short run. It is inescapable that the more decisions to prolong life are made, the fewer resources will be available to the other patients in nursing homes.)

The moral consensus on terminal care is much broader than that on abortion. No major religion in the United States is committed to an absolute position, and there is general agreement that wherever they are known, the patient's desires should be followed.[3] Congress recently built on this agreement in the Patient Self-Determination Act (PSDA), which requires hospitals, nursing homes, home health agencies, and health maintenance organizations to ask each entering patient whether he or she has completed an advanced directive (either a living will or the designation of an appropriate agent) expressing his or her wishes about treatment in situations in which he or she is no longer able to express an opinion.[4] It also requires the institutions to document the existence of an advance directive in the patient's record and to abide by the patient's wishes expressed through an advance directive. Finally, it requires the institutions to provide written information about advanced directives to patients and to conduct education for their staffs and communities. Obviously, the PSDA was written to eliminate the problems Dr. Hilfiker faced, and if Ms. Toivonen had responded to the nursing home's request, his decisions would have been simplified.

Four serious issues remain now that the PSDA has been passed and implemented: helping patients and families reach decisions, dealing with situations in which the patient's will is ambiguous or unknown, supporting caregivers who repeatedly face the problem Dr. Hilfiker and Ginger did, and maintaining the moral consensus.[5]

The first problem is to get people to make decisions and complete the written records necessary to implement the PSDA. Decisions about the end of life are difficult, and people tend to put them off. Few people entering an institution are prepared to address the question of appropriate terminal care.[6] A living will or a durable power of attorney designating an agent is desirable. The documentation should be clear and precise, and the patient's signature must be witnessed by people other than the next of kin who might have a financial stake in the outcome.

Beyond clear presentation of the medical facts, the institution should not influence patients' decisions, but it can either promote or discourage completion of the forms. If it takes a deliberately neutral stance, fewer forms will be completed than if it encourages completion. The best way to encourage completion might be to have the patient's attending physician explain the use of the forms and answer the patient's questions. However, doctors historically have been reluctant to raise the subject.[7] They might need training and encouragement to do so, and many might prefer that a hospital or nursing home employee be trained for the task. The questions of the institutional role versus the physician's role must be resolved if patients are to get satisfactory support.

The second problem is the remaining ambiguity. There will always be cases that do not exactly fit the law. For example, some patients might decline to sign the document but might or might not indicate their intentions in other ways. Others might be legally incompetent at the time of admission or become incompetent before the document can be signed. Some patients or their next of kin might bring a document from home later in the stay. What if this document looks inadequate or suspicious? What if the patient announces that she has changed her mind? What if his competence is fading, or if she can no longer speak but by gestures and actions seems to have changed her mind? As a general rule, the treatment should be continued when a reasonable doubt exists about the patient's desire, but these issues bring back Dr. Hilfiker's dilemma essentially unchanged.

Third, limited care is a new concept, and the quality of limited care will require new standards. The moral implications of the limitation of care quickly become entwined with the legal and public relations aspects. It is important that the family leaves content that the institution and its staff have helped in both medical and emotional senses. Anger or a sense of betrayal by the institution will make a volatile combination with their bereavement and possible feelings of guilt from the death. The caregivers must give emotional support to the family as well as to the patient. The problems of terminal care are emotionally demanding for the caregivers. They will provide better quality if they are supported in their efforts.

Fourth, extending the problem of relations with the individual families to the population at large, the institution can support and extend the moral consensus by effective and sensitive handling of the PSDA. The PSDA and the moral consensus behind it have one moral and several nonmoral benefits. Morally, they preserve what some believe is a central freedom of American life, the right to refuse medical care. Nonmorally, they allow choices that are less expensive for society than an absolute rule for the preservation of life and avoid the confrontational politics that have characterized the abortion debate. The limited demand for absolutism seems to arise among people who are remote from Dr. Hilfiker's reality. Outside the health care industry, it must be difficult to understand that until our lifetimes, Ms. Toivonen would have died from the pneumonia that followed her stroke three years ago. She expired as a personality with the initial stroke, and she survives as a biological mechanism only by technology. Dr. Hilfiker faces an array of choices that do not include any possibility of restoring her to conscious interaction with the world.

There are growing numbers of such cases, resulting from strokes, head injuries, birth injuries, and certain infectious diseases. It is part of the job of the health care industry to make the facts clear. These include both a candid description of these patients' condition and prognosis and an emphasis on the possibilities of prevention. Cigarette smoking, seat belts, alcohol abuse, poor prenatal care, and a lack of immunizations predispose the conditions that put people in Ms. Toivonen's position. It is our job to see that the possibilities of prevention are understood. Then some of the energies that go to advocating absolutist responses could be directed to avoiding the problem.

Thus one result of the PSDA is to relieve Dr. Hilfiker, at least in some cases, but to put the social version of his problem on the desk of every hospital or nursing home manager.

What should the institution do? If its leadership is opposed to the concept of self-determination, it will do only the minimum the law requires. But if it is in favor of the concept, it will work to make each patient and family satisfied with their choice, maximize the number of advance directives, and support its clinical personnel both in carrying out the intent of the directives and in dealing with ambiguous situations. This support implies the following managerial steps:

1. The resolution of the appropriate roles of employees and attending physicians
2. Discussion and clarification for personnel to make understanding and support of the PSDA as strong and widespread as possible, including a strong affirmation of patients' rights not to sign
3. The provision of explanatory material, education, and counseling services to patients (and possibly staff) on request
4. The training of admission personnel and support for them and clinical personnel dealing with ambiguous cases
5. The development of preventive programs that minimize the risk of a long period in a severely impaired or vegetative state like Ms. Toivonen's
6. The consideration of new patterns of care such as hospices, bereavement counseling, and religious support for patients and families who want them

7. The consideration of the rights of employees who might feel they cannot honor a living will request

The ethics committee is a proven device for dealing with these matters. It has two major roles, to identify and help solve any logistical and system problems that have ethical content and to assist patients, families, and caregivers in ambiguous or difficult cases.[8] In its first role, it develops information, sponsors debate, and reviews procedures and criteria to solve problems like the PSDA implementation. PSDA procedures, like any others, are developed and promulgated by the usual nonmoral mechanism. The individuals and committees developing them should be sensitive to the moral consequences. The ethics committee can review the result for moral implications. In its second role, the committee usually works with individuals to resolve ambiguities and to make them aware of the facts and their choices. It rarely judges individual cases, and it does not prescribe or assume a specific ethical stance beyond the basic right of a competent patient to choice.

Transplants (Case 7)

The most demanding problems of competing *prima facie* obligations tend to occur at the margins of experience, where life is tenuous, for example, or where procedures are new and untested. The prevailing U.S. consensus seems to be in favor of the liberal use of transplants and other very expensive technology. This premise is far from inevitable. Oregon has decided against certain transplants and other very costly treatments as Medicaid policy, for example, and frequencies are much lower in other advanced countries.[9]

Can we find ways in which the organization can help in the effective use of high technology? The criteria for distributing the transplants remains a moral question on which there is little consensus, as the article shows. Philosophically, the question is one of distributional equity, similar to, and some would say no more important than, questions about the regressivity of taxation or the eligibility for welfare benefits. The principle debates at the individual patient level are over whether factors other than the chance of success (such as whether the parents are married, whether a previous relationship with the patient has been established, or whether the patient's illness comes from self-abuse by smoking or drinking) should be considered.[10] There is also concern that race affects the likelihood of a given patient's receiving a transplant.[11] Within each transplanting institution there is an ethics-committee-like panel that tries to ensure consistency in the moral decisions that institution reaches. There are questions whether each institution should have full freedom to decide these issues as well as debates about the possible answers.

Once the institution has answered the allocation question, the remaining problems are nonmoral. They include

1. enhancing the supply of organs by encouraging donation (the donation process, called *harvesting*, involves emergency services and personnel who are not involved in transplants, the ethics of harvesting—when and from whom—seem to be a matter of agreement);[12]
2. maintaining the harvesting logistics, which require prompt, integrated actions by several different teams;
3. improving the national registry, to allow each participating institution equal access;
4. balancing the number of transplant sites with the supply of organs (success rates appear to be related to the volumes achieved by the teams);
5. supporting the staff against the stresses involved; and
6. supporting patients and their families.

The modern health care organization has nonmoral procedures to enhance these operations. Efforts to improve subordinate-superior relationships, consultation requirements, procedure guidelines, committees for consensus-building, and services for assisting the front-line personnel (such as personal counseling, relief time, and generally supportive management) will be effective here as they are in other organized activity. In transplant hospitals, these efforts can increase the probability of transplant success. Other hospitals need to address the issues as well, particularly as they relate to organ harvesting. Donor site hospitals can increase the success of organ harvesting, permitting a larger number of transplants.

A Theory for Dealing with *Prima Facie* Conflicts

Required assumptions about moral obligations

As these cases show, a general system of good management that promotes quality and efficiency will help resolve conflicting *prima facie* obligations. But inevitably, serious moral conflicts will remain. Can the organization help its members to deal with these as well? To a limited extent, the answer is yes, but to do so requires a consensus on certain assumptions about theories of moral obligation. By admitting the reality of the dilemmas posed in the cases, most of us implicitly accept a set of broadly held moral values. Two of these are essential to an organized effort to improve moral decisions. The first is Kant's imperative and a related set of utilitarian teleology sometimes described as universalism. Kant's axiom can be restated as,

> Act only on that maxim through which you can at the same time will that it should become universal law.[13]

In other words, Kant's principle requires that you act so that if any individual involved in the action were to be replaced by any other individual (a competing party, yourself, or one who was not previously involved), the action remains appropriate. This framing makes more clear the relation of Kant's precept to equity or justice. We will call it the principle of justice. For example, justice requires that the entire field of organ transplant candidates be considered if anyone is considered, and justice requires that all individuals have an equal opportunity to gain access to health care.

Strictly speaking, the Kantian principle does not create an obligation to transplant the organ rather than to leave it in the donor. To make rules for resolving specific *prima facie* conflicts, we will need another principle, which we state as,

> It is the obligation of health care organizations to promote wellness and well-being to the extent they are able.

We will call this the principle of beneficence. Here again, one might expect widespread acceptance, but because the organization must operate in a zone of public consensus, the principles must be carefully worded to stay within the limits.

These two principles, beneficence and justice, are broadly acceptable and consistent with the traditions of health care. They can form the basis of a set of further rules for dealing with *prima facie* conflicts, beyond the duty of being efficient and effective as a manager.

Guiding the organization's *prima facie* selections

In the final analysis, choices between conflicting *prima facie* obligations are made only by individuals. But in modern organizations, individuals frequently act in concert, both explicitly, as when a committee votes, and implicitly, when one member relies on the actions of another.

Recognizing the limits of authority and the need to work within a public consensus, let us try to formulate some guidelines that might promote sound selections.

Avoiding the banality of evil. The first step under the assumptions of beneficence and justice is an obligation to examine all questions for their moral implications. It appears that many serious moral errors occur simply because no one stopped to think of the consequences. Unfortunately this tendency seems more prominent when those consequences befall an individual or group who is disadvantaged or considered inferior. Hannah Arendt noted that Eichmann, the German officer who supervised wholesale slaughter of Jews, seemed at his trial not so much deliberately evil as unquestioning, a passive rather than active participant in a scene of unspeakable horror. She called this tendency "the banality of evil."[14] The banality of evil has been noted many times, among people with the best of intentions. It often arises when people are careless, incompletely trained, poorly motivated, or overworked. Ignorance, haste, fatigue, and insensitivity make it possible to overlook the full set of consequences. So, of course, does an organizational culture that denies or suppresses the implications of corporate actions in the name of profit, financial necessity, or meeting goals.

The organization that aspires to be beneficent and just must overcome these pressures. It must encourage its members to stop and consider whether a proposed action uses any group or individual as a means rather than an end. This consideration requires a deliberate, active review, with extra emphasis on the impact of the action on those who might normally be overlooked. Overcoming the banality of evil might be the most important step in dealing with *prima facie* obligations. It might be that the unrecognized and therefore neglected opportunities, the sins of omission, are more serious in total than the incorrect choices from recognized lists.

Developing moral consideration of process. A second step is to examine management processes that are identified as having serious moral implications. The processes must themselves meet the tests of beneficence and justice; that is, they should encourage broad participation, honesty, full information, and a dispassionate arena appropriate to the question. Physician privileging and all individual employment decisions fall in this group. Budgeting and staffing decision processes must be examined. A principal purpose of the examination is to encourage people to "put their moral glasses on," to view the proposal from perspectives other than their own. Like with the authority to command, it soon becomes clear that under the assumptions of beneficence and justice, the processes for sound moral judgement are an extension of those for sound nonmoral judgement. The criteria for good processes are expanded more than they are changed.

Listing the prima facie obligations and evaluating the theory supporting each. It is helpful to begin a specific selection among prima facie alternatives by listing the various obligations and identifying to whom they are held and under what theory of obligations. It is important to be as comprehensive as possible in identifying the obligations. An overlooked obligation can only accidentally be honored. In general, health care managers are likely to encounter obligations to the same groups: patients and their families, physicians and employees, the institution or organization, the community or society, and self and family. The list is an aid to avoid oversights.

Identifying the theory supporting each obligation helps clarify its importance. Certain obligations superficially seem to have more support than they do under scrutiny. The obligation of the referees to the rapist physician is one of these; there seems to be a tendency to think of former colleagues as deserving of some special consideration that a strict reading of Kant forbids (unless the doctors believed that the recipients of the letters would have no interest in the existence of a rape conviction). In particular, the Hippocratic oath contains a suggestion that loyalty to physicians should supersede all else. The first paragraph begins, "I will look upon him who taught me this art even as one of my parents,... [and] regard his offspring as my own brethren." This seems consistent with a vague but popular loyalty to one's relatives, ethnic group, or close associates. Only a little reflection on the consequences of this rule casts doubt on its beneficence as well as its justice. The question, How loyal I should be to a convicted rapist? is only one concern. Another is that in today's mobile society, I might have as great an obligation to people I might sometime know as those I once knew. A third is that Kant wisely and deliberately did not differentiate classes of humanity, even for blood relatives.

Identifying alternative solutions. Just as many moral problems begin with the banality of evil, many others are caused by inflexible pursuit of a specific solution. Reviewing and expanding the list of alternatives are often fruitful. The referee doctors, like most people writing reference letters, had several options they could have pursued, including that they did not feel his conviction should be held against him, for various reasons. Dr. Lapin's actions in the DRG case are based on an overly narrow assumption; he should have made several alternative ones.

Identifying alternative solutions, like identifying the full list of obligations, is an inductive process. That is, it calls for the synthesis of new actions from the available information. Inductive thinking may be more difficult than deduction, which describes most rule-following kinds of logic. It is improved by

- professional competence, that is, a complete mastery of the technology and its opportunities;
- communication of ideas (two heads are better than one);
- accurate and complete fact bases, implying good and accessible records; and
- practice, because cases generate results, hints, or even principles that carry forward to subsequent cases.

A large part of management lies behind these characteristics, including selection and credentialing, employee satisfaction and retention, information systems, and organizational cultures that empower employees and encourage communication.

The imagination and flexibility with which alternatives are sought is a test of management skill, another part of the moral challenge of management. Good managers are adept at finding solutions that allow all parties to thrive. They build organizations that select good people and encourage them to get better. Like many other management arts, this one is developed over time, by practice.

Evaluating the potential benefit and harm of the alternative solutions. The first objective of the management process is to reach a quick, correct solution to as many cases as possible, while identifying the difficult ones for more elaborate treatment. Particularly in the easy cases, identification and evaluation occur simultaneously. Ideas are uncovered, tested against the facts and moral principles, and quickly discarded or pursued. Inevitably, some taxing and stressful cases remain. In those cases more formal methods might reach the best decision while minimizing the stress to the individuals involved.

Sometimes there is no good solution. When this occurs, it is necessary to consider the lesser of evils, or the least worst solution. Using both approaches is often helpful. The search for the least worst allows one to eliminate the obviously inferior alternatives and reduce the list to a few acceptable ones. When the right act remains unclear, the most important action is to double check the possibilities for alternative solutions, if possible by bringing in more consultants and assistants.

Applying the rules for managing conflicting obligations to clinical areas

Three of the cases involve clinical decisions, and in real life a larger proportion of the troublesome issues have at least clinical components. The fact that clinical professionals are involved does not exempt management; the moral obligations under rules of utilitarian beneficence and justice parallel the legal ones now common in malpractice. Neither should the process be different, but obviously it must be clinically as well as morally informed.

The evaluative process is initially deductive. That is, it proceeds from a set of facts to an accepted principle to an inescapable conclusion. An example is the syllogism, Ms. Jones is terminally ill with cancer. We should not use expensive chemotherapy when it cannot affect the outcome. Therefore, Ms. Jones should not receive chemotherapy. This logic is useful as far as it goes, but medical ethicists note that it is simplistic, inflexible, and unsatisfying in the face of the richness and variety of real medical practice. (Suppose, for example, that Ms. Jones' daughter is engaged, and chemotherapy would allow a few weeks of relative health, during which Ms. Jones could attend the wedding.) Graber and Thomasma trace a series of steps by which the deductive syllogism is expanded to the ongoing consideration of both facts and principle leading to a flexible, individualized evaluation without sacrificing either objectivity or the moral principle. Their approach relies heavily on principles and rules derived from prior experience.[15] It would evaluate an array of alternatives, developed by induction, against a multidimensional scale that includes both a humane evaluation of Ms. Jones's needs and the social need to control the cost of expensive therapies.

The problem in designing such complex evaluative systems is to maintain rigor while encouraging flexibility and innovation. It is easy at the deductive extreme to be insensitive and rigid, but it is equally easy for the more complex approaches to deteriorate into ad hoc or even purely subjective solutions. Graber and Thomasma introduce the notion of virtue (which we will address in Part IV), the skill, habit, or predisposition of the professional to be beneficent and just, and go beyond that to note that the clinical practice of medicine intrinsically involves ethical thinking. They argue that:

> (1) A merely deductive medical ethics would be inadequate because much more complex reasoning is required to resolve problems, and (2) medical ethics is not just applied normative ethics but also a branch of medicine itself.... Both diagnosis and therapeutics involve values, however, values that may conflict among themselves or among others. Some of these values are ethical. As a result, decisions to be made must take all these values into account if medical ethics is to be properly understood.[16]

Much the same could be said of health care management. Its purpose is to influence the delivery of health care in ways that inevitably involve values. The manager's decisions must take these values into account together with technical ones if health care management is to be properly understood. The important issue for managers is not how to decide who gets the scarce organ or the intensive care unit bed, it is how to help others make the decisions and to see that the supply of beds and organs is adequate. The recommended processes begin with a sound scientific and factual foundation and expand on it to meet the gravity of the problem. They draw on teams such as ethics committees, rather than individuals, to ensure that no relevant issue is left unexamined and no viewpoint denied a hearing. They use carefully developed and formally ratified procedures to assure consistency. They take pains to avoid prejudice on any grounds, treating each individual as equal to the next in all respects not explicitly addressed in the criteria. They include formal mechanisms to evaluate the consequences of each alternative and to find new alternatives. In the end, they leave the decision to a few identified individuals whose right or obligation it is to decide. And they recognize the demands that have been made on these individuals and assist them with the consequences of the stress.

Ethics committees and counseling assistance play an important role here. A second opinion often both improves the judgment and relieves the caregiver. It is important to note that the line supervisor is the most common source of counsel. Thus a good organization trains its supervisors, especially its clinical managers, to help with the typical moral problems their subordinates face.

Without question, these procedures are superior to others that omit or diminish these steps. One task of health care managers is to see that they are followed throughout a bureaucratic organization that might involve several thousand members. That, of course, is a nonmoral process that begins with the relationship between the doctor or the employee and the hospital. When that relationship is collaborative and synergistic, rather than competitive, the foundation has been laid.[17]

Notes

1. H. Mintzberg, *The Nature of Managerial Work* (New York: Harper & Row, 1973).
2. W. E. Deming, *Out of the Crisis* (Cambridge, MA: Massachusetts Institute of Technology, 1986).
3. President's Commission for the Study of Ethical Problems in Medicine and Biomedical and Behavioral Research, *Deciding to Forego Life-Sustaining Treatment* (Washington, DC: U.S. Government Printing Office, 1983).
4. Part of the Omnibus Budget Reconciliation Act of 1990, Pub. L. 101-508.
5. Hastings Center, "Practicing the PSDA," Special Supplement, *Hastings Center Report* 21, no. 5 (September–October 1991): S1–S16.
6. E. R. Gamble, P. J. McDonald, and P. R. Lichtstein, "Knowledge, Attitudes, and Behavior or Elderly Persons Regarding Living Wills," *Archives of Internal Medicine* 151, no. 2 (February 1991): 277–80.
7. L. L. Brunetti, S. D. Carperos, and R. E. Westlund, "Physicians' Attitudes Towards Living Wills and Cardiopulmonary Resuscitation," *Journal of General Internal Medicine* 6, no. 4 (July–August 1991): 323–29.
8. American Hospital Association, *Report of the Special Committee on Biomedical Ethics* (Chicago: The Association, 1985), 33–35.
9. H. G. Welch, and E. B. Larsen, "Dealing with Limited Resources: Oregon's Decision to Curtail Funding for Organ Transplants," *New England Journal of Medicine* 319, no. 3 (1984): 171–73.
10. M. Durbin, "Bone Marrow Transplantation: Economic, Ethical, and Social Issues," *Pediatrics* 82, no. 5 (November 1988): 774–83.
11. P. J. Held, M. V. Pauly, R. R. Bovberg, et al. "Access to Kidney Transplantation. Has the United States Eliminated Income and Racial Differences?" *Archives of Internal Medicine* 148, no. 12 (December 1988): 2594–600.
12. A. Grenvik, "Ethical Dilemmas in Organ Donation and Transplantation," *Critical Care Medicine* 16, no. 10 (October 1988): 1012–18; also M. Durbin, "Bone Marrow Transplantation: Economic, Ethical, and Social Issues," *Pediatrics* 82, no. 5 (November 1988): 774–83.
13. B. Aune, *Kant's Theory of Morals* (Princeton, NJ: Princeton University Press, 1979), 112.
14. H. Arendt, *Eichmann in Jerusalem: A Report on the Banality of Evil* (New York: Viking Press, 1965).
15. G. C. Graber, and D. C. Thomasma, *Theory and Practice in Medical Ethics* (New York: Continuum Publishing Co., 1989).
16. Ibid., 176.
17. J. R. Griffith, *The Well-Managed Community Hospital* (Ann Arbor: Health Administration Press, 1987), 379–430.

Part IV
Improving Virtue

Case 8

The Question of Venial Sins

The following are commonly encountered personal temptations for managers that illustrate the concepts of virtue. These are issues for which almost everyone's theory of moral obligations offers a clear answer, and for most it is difficult to imagine serious *prima facie* conflicts. Yet they are also situations that are often handled incorrectly. For some of the more complex issues, the question is not the selection of right versus wrong so much as good versus better. That is, we can all agree on a satisfactory solution, but one can envision other possibilities that are better.

The concept of promoting virtue, of being a morally good person, begins with an understanding of the temptations and of the ways to build stronger responses. The question to consider is not so much, What should be done? as it is, How do you build an organization where more people do the best thing?

The following are personal and professional moral issues that have sometimes damaged organizations and hampered individual careers.

   A. Employees are presented with a number of questionable material offers, including the following:
   1. Gifts from suppliers
   2. Gifts, entertainment, and free medical care from attending physicians
   3. Special treatment from other employees, e.g., your spouse is hospitalized (Although you know the hospital's fringe benefits do not cover the full cost of hospitalization, no bill materializes.)

4. Special treatment from trustees, e.g., the bank that handles hospital's accounts and that is prominently represented on the board unexplainably offers you a mortgage at a rate 2 percent below the competition

B. Managerial employees have an employment contract that is less explicit than it looks. Here are some questions often not spelled out in advance:
1. On what terms may you accept additional employment or volunteer for community activities?
2. Who has rights to property of value developed on company time (e.g., a computer program)?
3. What constitutes a full day's work for an executive?

C. Extending the issues of the management's employment contract, here are some issues for which the organization's rights are prescribed by law or custom but for which a virtuous manager might perceive an additional obligation:
1. Alcoholism and substance abuse
2. Anxiety and stress
3. Overweight
4. Smoking
5. Sexual life style
   a. Moral issues (over and above those involved in any sexual liaison) raised by sexual relations with superiors or subordinates
   b. Sexual preference
   c. Marriage to an individual in the same organization
   d. Timing of pregnancy

Case 9

Dr. Burt of St. Elizabeth's

Introductory Note: Hospitals deal routinely with the stuff of tragedy: the beginning of life, the end of life, the foreshortening or impairment of life by accident or disease. As a result, their moral failures can easily become tragedies themselves. What in other industries is merely unfortunate or painful can be disastrous in health care. At root in the Dr. Burt case and in the Dr. Billig case that follows are several moral failures that occur more frequently than any of us would like to admit. In each case, the failures interacted to make a disaster.

The highest moral challenge of health care managers is to understand what these failures are, why they occur, and how to take deliberate action to avoid them. What formal and informal steps must be taken to see that physicians' privileges are appropriate to their skills and that their practice does not exceed the privilege limitations? And how does the manager promote an organization that takes these steps habitually, automatically, and invariably?

Charges Against Doctor Bring Ire and Questions[*]

by Isabel Wilkerson

Dayton, Ohio, Dec. 9—Relief, shame and anger were being expressed today in this central Ohio city where for 22 years

---

[*]*The New York Times*, 11 December 1988, sec. I p. 32. Copyright © 1988 by The New York Times Company. Reprinted by permission.

Dr. James C. Burt performed what experts say was crude experimentation on hundreds of women without their consent.

This week the Ohio State Medical Board formally charged Dr. Burt with "gross immorality" and "grossly unprofessional conduct" in surgery he performed to restructure his patients' genitals, procedures that the board said often caused permanent physical damage. Dr Burt, who is still practicing out of his office here, has 30 days to request a hearing, which could be scheduled as early as next month.

The doctor, who detailed some of his procedures in a 1975 book, did not return phone calls to his office this week. But he has said in recent months that he was confident he would be vindicated.

In Dayton, many people are relieved that charges have been brought against Dr. Burt by the medical board. But heartbroken patients here and incredulous physicians elsewhere are trying to figure out why it took so long for his practices to attract the scrutiny of medical investigators and wonder whether other doctors are trying out unproven techniques on their patients.

Colleagues kept silent, board says

In all of the soul-searching and fingerpointing, the state medical board is now looking into the role and responsibility of his colleagues who, board officials say, silently watched as many of Dr. Burt's patients suffered permanent physical damage.

"There is a great deal of concern about the breakdown in the reporting system," said Lauren Lubow, an attorney and spokesman for the board. "The doctors in the Dayton medical community are under investigation for what they knew."

Janet Phillips went to Dr. Burt with complaints of cramps six years ago and was one of hundreds of patients who ended up with her anatomy changed. "You're raised to trust your minister, your policeman and your doctor," she said. "He was the one with the degree on the wall. He knew medicine better than I did. I didn't think he would hurt me."

Physicians across the country said they were astonished and outraged that Dr. Burt had operated outside recognized standards for so long. "It's a disgrace to all of medicine," said Dr. Sidney M. Wolfe, an internist who is director of the Public Citizens' Health Research Group, a consumer advocacy group. "His procedures were several standard deviations from what is acceptable. And only now are people who should have spoken up 20 years ago slowly, timidly coming out of the closet."

Experts on medical ethics say that the complicity appeared widespread. "If hundreds of women underwent a useless and dangerous medical procedure without explicit consent, then anyone who stood by and did not bring it to the attention of the medical board or the hospital trustees or the women who had the procedure was behaving unethically," said Dr. Arthur Caplan, director of the Center for Biomedical Ethics at the University of Minnesota.

Surgery prohibited

The procedure has not been performed since January 1987. Last month, the board prohibited Dr. Burt from performing any surgery pending its investigation, but it has not revoked his license.

Dr. Burt, once a well-regarded physician considered merely eccentric, began the special surgery in 1966. Explaining his philosophy in his 1975 book, "Surgery of Love," Dr. Burt wrote: "Women are structurally inadequate for intercourse. This is a pathological condition amenable to surgery." In franker terms, he also said that his surgery would turn women into "horny little mice" and asserted that "the difference between rape and rapture is salesmanship."

In the book, which he financed himself, Dr. Burt admitted to performing reconstructive surgery on "many hundreds" of women without their consent, usually after the birth of a child. "The patient," he wrote, "had not been informed that anything more had been done to her than delivery and episiotomy and repair, or 'Yes, you had stitches with your delivery.'"

The surgery often included removing the hood of a patient's clitoris, repositioning the vagina, moving the urethra, and altering the walls between the rectum and vagina. It was intended, the doctor wrote, to redesign the vagina to increase sexual responsiveness.

Instead, the surgery caused sexual dysfunction, extensive scarring, chronic infections of the kidney, bladder and vagina and the need for corrective surgery in many patients, according to the Ohio State Medical Board. Although some of the patients have expressed satisfaction with their surgery, at least one patient suffered phlebitis, blood clots and a heart attack, the board said, and several have permanent disabilities.

The procedure is not recognized by the American College of Obstetricians and Gynecologists, the standard-setting organization for gynecology, nor taught in American medical schools.

Gynecologists have told one former patient, Cheryl Sexton, that corrective surgery will require four specialists—a urologist, a neurologist, a plastic surgeon and gynecologist—and will cost $25,000.

Dr. Burt, who did not return repeated telephone calls to his office this week, told The Dayton Daily News on Nov. 20 that the criticisms came from "dissatisfied women who may have had complications, who may be lying, who may have had positive feelings turn negative when forced to pay the bill and women who stand to make a lot of money from the lies."

Dr. Burt began his medical career in 1945 when he graduated from the University of Rochester Medical School and held his internship at the Baylor College of Medicine in Houston immediately thereafter. He did his residency at the Lying-in Hospital at the University of Chicago and the Sloan Hospital of the Columbia Presbyterian Medical Center from 1949 to 1951.

He is neither a fellow of the American College of Obstetricians and Gynecologists, the professional organization that includes 90 percent of gynecologists, nor certified by the American Board of Obstetrics and Gynecology.

Mrs. Phillips was one of the many women who went to Dr. Burt for a relatively minor physical problem, in her case cramps. She was told she needed a hysterectomy because her Fallopian tubes were "rotting."

She ended up with a changed anatomy and suffers chronic infections, extreme difficulty urinating and excruciating pain if she attempts intercourse. The strain eventually destroyed her marriage, which ended in divorce five years ago, she said.

Seven hours of surgery completely changed her life. "I feel like a freak," Mrs. Phillips said. "I can't date. I can't ride horses. I can't urinate like normal women. I was sexually abused by Dr. Burt. He stole parts of my body."

Gynecologists knew about Dr. Burt's surgery and recognized his work when they examined his former patients. "Doctors would say, 'Dr. Burt's done surgery on you, hasn't he?' or 'Have you been to see Dr. Burt?'" said Joy Martin, who had to get corrective surgery after Dr. Burt delivered her son in 1974.

Mrs. Phillips and Mrs. Sexton have filed lawsuits, seeking $6 million, against Dr. Burt and St. Elizabeth's Hospital, where he performed most of his surgeries. Thirty-five other former patients are expected to file lawsuits in the next few weeks, said Lee Sambol, the lawyer for the women. Ten previous malpractice lawsuits against Dr. Burt over the past 12 years were dropped when other physicians refused to testify.

"We've all had Dr. Burt's patients, and we've tried to undo the work he has done," said Dr. Robert Hilty, a gynecologist who was chairman of the Department of Obstetrics and Gynecology at Kettering Medical Center in Dayton for 18 years. "But we need the freedom to openly criticize without fear of legal retribution."

Some doctors say they repeatedly told investigators from the Ohio State Medical Board about Dr. Burt's eccentricities, but say the board did not take action until Gov. Richard Celeste wrote the board about the case.

Doctor Gives Up Medical License In Face of 'Love Surgery' Hearings*

Columbus, Ohio, Jan. 26 (AP)—Dr. James C. Burt, a gynecologist facing 41 violations of medical ethics involving his self-described "love surgery" on female genitalia, has surrendered his license to practice medicine.

The State Medical Board said Wednesday that it had accepted Dr. Burt's offer to surrender his Ohio medical license. It said the action included a requirement that the 67-year-old physician not practice medicine anywhere in the country.

In a statement, Dr. Burt denied that he had ever performed the surgery without patient consent. The surgery involved a physical alteration of female genitalia intended to enhance sexual responsiveness.

"Every patient I have ever delivered or operated upon has had at least one informed consent," said Dr. Burt, who practiced in Dayton.

Board cited patients' problems

Last month, the medical board charged him with "gross immorality" for 41 alleged violations ranging from overprescribing drugs to performing unnecessary surgeries. The board charged that the operation

---

*The New York Times, 27 January 1989, p. A16. Reprinted with the permission of The Associated Press.

100 Improving Virtue

Figure IV.1 Hospitals Serving Dayton, Ohio, 1987

Hospital, Address, Telephone, Administrator, Approval and Facility Codes, Multihospital System	Classification Codes				Facilities	Inpatient Data				Newborn Data		Expense (thousands of dollars)			Personnel
	Control	Service	Stay			Beds	Admissions	Census	Occupancy (percent)	Bassinets	Births	Total	Payroll	
★ American Hospital Association (AHA) membership ☐ Joint Commission on Accreditation of Healthcare Organizations (JCAHO) accreditation + American Osteopathic Hospital Association (AOHA) membership ○ American Osteopathic Association (AOA) accreditation △ Commission on Accreditation of Rehabilitation Facilities (CARF) accreditation Control codes 61, 63, 64, 71, 72 and 73 indicate hospitals listed by AOHA, but not registered by AHA. For definition of numerical codes, see page A20														
DAYTON — Montgomery County														
⊞ CHILDREN'S MEDICAL CENTER, One Children's Plaza, Zip 45404; tel. 513/226-8300 Laurence P. Harkness, President & Chief Executive Officer **A1**a 3 5 9 10 **F1** 3 5 6 10 12 14 15 16 22 23 24 26 28 31 34 35 38 41 42 43 44 45 46 47 51 53 54	23	50	S		139	6190	105	75.5	0	0	40784	19628	872
☐ DARTMOUTH HOSPITAL, 1038 Salem Ave., Zip 45406; tel. 513/278-7917 George Chopivsky, Chief Executive Officer; Judy Wortham, Associate Administrator **A1**a 10 **F**24 28 29 30 31 32 34 42 49	33	22	S		38	510	32	84.2	0	0	5369	2365	109
DAYTON MENTAL HEALTH CENTER, 2611 Wayne Ave., Zip 45420; tel. 513/258-0440 Patricia A. Torvik Ph.D., Superintendent **A**9 10 **F**19 24 30 42 46 47	12	22	L		402	1118	302	75.1	0	0	23479	14518	609
⊞ GOOD SAMARITAN HOSPITAL AND HEALTH CENTER, 2222 Philadelphia Dr., Zip 45406; tel. 513/278-2612 K. Douglas Deck, President & Chief Executive Officer **A1**a 2 3 5 8 9 10 **F1** 2 3 4 5 6 7 8 9 10 11 12 14 15 16 20 23 24 26 27 28 29 30 31 32 34 35 36 40 41 42 44 45 46 47 48 49 51 53 54 **S**5115	21	10	S		560	21963	409	73.0	24	1923	111915	51860	2226
★ ○ GRANDVIEW HOSPITAL AND MEDICAL CENTER (Includes Southview Hospital And Family Health Center, 1997 Miamisburg-Centerville Rd., Zip 45459, tel. 513/439-6000 Michael J. Setty, Senior Vice President & Administrator), 405 Grand Ave., Zip 45405; tel. 513/226-3200 Richard J. Minor, President & Chief Executive Officer **A**9 10 11 12 13 **F1** 2 3 4 6 10 11 12 14 15 16 20 21 23 24 26 27 30 31 32 34 35 36 37 40 44 45 46 47 50 52 53 54	23	10	S		452	12812	257	56.9	35	800	78170	31813	1431
⊞ △ MIAMI VALLEY HOSPITAL, One Wyoming St., Zip 45409; tel. 513/223-6192 Thomas G. Breitenbach, President & Chief Executive Officer **A1**a 2 3 5 7 8 9 10 **F1** 2 3 4 5 6 7 8 9 10 11 13 15 16 17 20 22 23 24 25 26 27 28 29 30 31 33 34 35 36 37 38 40 42 43 44 45 46 47 48 49 50 51 53 54 SOUTHVIEW HOSPITAL AND FAMILY HEALTH CENTER See Grandview Hospital And Medical Center	23	10	S		731	22960	486	66.5	44	3969	138521	59850	2329
⊞ △ ST. ELIZABETH MEDICAL CENTER, 601 Edwin C Moses Blvd., Zip 45408; tel. 513/229-6000 James B. Makos, Acting President (Total facility includes 30 beds in nursing home-type unit) **A1**a 2 3 5 7 8 9 10 **F1** 3 4 5 6 7 8 9 10 11 12 14 15 16 19 20 23 24 25 26 27 30 31 32 33 34 35 36 37 38 40 41 42 44 46 52 53 54 **S**1485	21	10	S	TF H	616 586	20008 19965	450 445	74.5 —	35 35	2358 2358	96538 95849	50527 50255	2275 —
⊞ VETERANS ADMINISTRATION MEDICAL CENTER, 4100 W. Third St., Zip 45428; tel. 513/268-6511 Alan G. Harper, Director (Total facility includes 959 beds in nursing home-type unit) **A1**a 3 5 8 **F1** 2 3 6 10 11 12 14 15 16 19 20 21 23 24 25 26 27 28 29 30 31 32 34 35 41 42 44 46 47 48 49 50 53 54	45	10	S	TF H	1499 540	11264 10623	1236 393	82.5 —	0 0	0 0	67434 49090	44269 31807	1714 1579

Source: Reprinted with permission from *American Hospital Association Guide to the Health Care Field* 1988 edition, copyright 1988 by the American Hospital Association, pp. A247–48.

caused sexual dysfunction, emotional distress, infection, chronic pain, incontinence and the need for corrective surgery in many patients.

At least three malpractice suits are pending against Dr. Burt, each asking $3 million in damages. The women involved say Dr. Burt performed the surgery without their consent.

He had faced a hearing Monday before the medical board, but the panel said it was no longer necessary since license revocation is the maximum penalty the board could impose.

Dr. Burt's lawyer, Earl Moore, said the doctor had been considering retirement for some time and did not believe the board would treat him fairly.

"He will write and lecture and give seminars," Mr. Moore said. "The saga of Doctor Burt is far from over."

Dr. Burt was brought to public attention when the CBS News show "West 57th" reported on his "female circumcision" technique. The procedure involved the reconstruction and relocation of the vagina and the removal of flesh covering the clitoris, an external tissue that responds to sexual stimulation. Dr. Burt described the technique in his 1975 book, "Surgery of Love."

Dr. Burt performed 170 of the operations at St. Elizabeth Medical Center in Dayton, the last one in February 1987. Hospital officials, who requested he stop the operations, said Tuesday that an investigation concluded that all 170 were done with patient consent.

Case 10

Commodore Quinn and Captain Hodges

Introductory Note: In effect, the decision of the appeals panel in the Billig case and the testimony of the trial reveal a double failing. First, the Bethesda Hospital organization privileged Dr. Billig in areas where, in retrospect, it should not have; and second, the Navy tried him incorrectly.

The key moral roles are played not by Billig, the legal target, but by his superiors, Captain Fletcher, Captain Hodges, and Commodore Quinn. The central questions are two: First, how could they have prevented or shortened the series of cardiovascular surgical deaths? Second, what might encourage the physicians managing Bethesda Naval Hospital to have acted better or faster?

Officer Asserts Efforts at Inquiry On Top Surgeon Were Thwarted*

by Philip M. Boffey

Washington, Jan. 15—A Navy hospital administrator testified today that his efforts to force an investigation of Comdr. Donal M. Billig, the former top heart surgeon at the Bethesda Naval Hospital, for questions of surgical incompetence and dishonesty were sharply

---

*The New York Times, 16 January 1986, sec. I, p. 18. Copyright © 1986 by The New York Times Company. Reprinted by permission.

criticized by superiors who accused him of trying to ruin the famed hospital's reputation.

The witness, Capt. Leon C. Hodges Jr., former executive officer at the hospital, was one of three people to testify today at a general court-martial in which Dr. Billig is charged with negligence that killed five patients and with dereliction of duty for performing 24 unsupervised coronary bypass operations at a time when his surgical privileges were supposedly limited to less complicated procedures.

Captain Hodges said that he was "really chewed out severely" by Commodore James J. Quinn because in October 1983 he temporarily took away Dr. Billig's credentials to perform heart surgery and initiated an internal investigation into Dr. Billig's performance.

"He accused me of ruining the reputation of an outstanding physician" and of "ruining a program at the Naval Medical Center," Captain Hodges said in describing a telephone call he received in October 1983 from Commodore Quinn. "To me, it was really a threat," he added.

Captain Hodges said two other officers had criticized his efforts to force a detailed investigation of Dr. Billig. He said one, Capt. J. Raymond Fletcher, former director of surgical services at the hospital, complained it "had taken years" to build up the cardiothoracic surgery program at Bethesda, and "this would get out and ruin the whole program."

Captain Hodges, who now commands a naval hospital in Philadelphia, also testified that another officer, Capt. Raymond B. Johnson, then commander at the Bethesda hospital, "was very annoyed at me for pushing this" and ordered him not to appear at a crucial hearing at which Dr. Billig's credentials to perform heart surgery were reinstated in November 1983.

Both Commodore Quinn and Captain Fletcher received letters of censure for their roles in the affair and left the Navy. Dr. Quinn is now the vice president for hospital operations at the New York University Medical Center.

Dr. Quinn, who testified earlier today, said he learned in March 1983 that Dr. Billig experienced professional problems in a previous job at the Monmouth Medical Center in Long Branch, N.J. He said he did not suspend Dr. Billig at the time because he did not consider him a danger to patients and because colleagues said he was a competent thoracic surgeon, although not yet a qualified heart surgeon. Instead, Dr. Quinn said he ordered an investigation.

However, Captain Hodges testified later that an investigation initiated at that time went so slowly it had not even been completed a year later, while another investigation begun after his effort to restrict Dr. Billig in October 1983 was so superficial that the investigator never got in touch with anyone at Monmouth Medical Center or other places Dr. Billig had worked.

A third witness, Dr. Cyril Arvantis, chairman of the surgery department at Monmouth Medical Center, testified that Dr. Billig had been expelled from the staff there in 1981 after an exhaustive investigation into a high rate of surgical complications.

He said he had told Bethesda hospital officials on the telephone that Dr. Billig "should not be permitted to join the Navy, be in the Navy, or operate in the Navy" but that his evaluation was treated with "aloof courtesy" and "that was the end of the conversation."

Surgeon Gashed Main Artery Of Patient, Navy Trial Is Told*

Washington, Jan. 25 (AP)—Dr. Donal M. Billig once slashed a patient's main artery and panicked as blood spurted from the three-quarter-inch gash, a witness testified Friday at the Navy surgeon's court-martial.

Another surgeon put his hand on the aorta to stop the bleeding, said Dr. Phyllis Ann Edwards, a lieutenant commander who is a general surgeon at Bethesda Naval Hospital. "He really was immobilized," she said of Commander Billig, recalling the November 1984 incident at the hospital.

The patient, Lois Parent, 41 years old, the wife of a Marine Corps officer, died in the operating room where she was undergoing surgery for replacement of the aortic valve. Dr. Edwards was the second assistant surgeon.

On trial in five deaths

Dr. Billig is charged with involuntary manslaughter in the deaths of Mrs. Parent and four other patients at Bethesda. He was dismissed last

---

*The New York Times, 26 January 1986, sec. I, p. 19. Reprinted with the permission of The Associated Press.

April as head of the cardiothoracic surgery unit at the hospital for what the Navy termed "an insufficient level of surgical competence."

Dr. Edwards said Dr. Billig approached the aorta from "the wrong plane." The aorta, which carries blood to all parts of the body, starts at the heart's left ventricle. Dr. Edwards said that when Dr. Billig exposed the outer skin of the aorta, an assisting surgeon, Dr. Charles Lee, warned him of the danger but Dr. Billig went ahead anyway.

"The aorta tore and blood spurted for 15 seconds," she said.

'Blood was filling the chest'

Dr. Lee put his hand on the ruptured aorta to control the bleeding, Dr. Edwards said. "The blood was just filling the chest," she said.

The surgeons connected Mrs. Parent to a heart-lung machine to stop the bleeding by cooling her body. The cooling took about an hour, while Dr. time Lee [sic] held his hand on the gash.

Dr. Billig then placed a graft on the artery, but, Dr. Edwards said in court Friday: "In sewing the graft, to illustrate his panic, he was sewing totally incorrectly. The suture was so tangled in the way he had done it, I asked if he wanted it done over."

She said he did not respond.

Lieut. Comdr. Michael Curreri of the prosecution panel, asked Dr. Edwards if Dr. Billig's panic was out of character. "No, I felt it was in character—I had seen it before," she said.

The trial resumes Monday when Dr. Lee is to testify.

Navy Surgeon's Conviction In Three Deaths Overturned*

by Philip M. Boffey

Washington, April 14—Comdr. Donal M. Billig, the former chief heart surgeon at the Bethesda Navy Hospital who was convicted two years ago of involuntary manslaughter and negligent homi-

---

*The New York Times, 15 April 1988, p. A17. Copyright © 1988 by The New York Times Company. Reprinted by permission.

cide in the deaths of three patients, was freed from confinement today after a military appeals court said it was not convinced he was guilty.

The Navy-Marine Corps Court of Military Review also said that the Navy surgeon, who was convicted in early 1986 after a highly publicized general court-martial, had been the victim of "a smear campaign" in which military prosecutors sought to portray him "as a bungling, one-eyed surgeon who should have known better than even to enter an operating room because of his past mistakes and poor eyesight."

"This tactic should not have been permitted by the military judge," the appeals court said, because it forced Dr. Billig to defend himself not only against the charges involving patients at Bethesda but "to explain and account for virtually all of his mistakes, professional setbacks, or surgical misadventures during the previous 20 years."

Dr. Billig was sentenced to four years in prison and began serving his sentence in March 1986.

The appeals court said that this "bad surgeon" theory put forth by the prosecutors "permeated the trial proceedings and undoubtedly influenced the court members' decisions."

In setting aside the conviction, the appeals court concluded that it was not satisfied beyond a reasonable doubt that Dr. Billig was guilty of any of the derelictions for which he was convicted. Dr. Billig also had been sentenced to dismissal from the service and forfeiture of all pay and allowances.

The court essentially found that the surgical procedures and techniques for which Dr. Billig had been condemned fell within medically accepted standards, and that some of the adverse medical outcomes for which he had been blamed may have been due to other causes.

Today's action was likely to be applauded by many doctors. Some medical authorities said at the time of the court-martial that criminal penalties for physicians would inhibit doctors from taking appropriate risks.

Earlier setbacks recalled

But prosecutors said the most egregious cases of medical negligence called for such penalties. Sanctions against doctors generally range from civil lawsuits to censure by state boards to loss of license.

The charges against Dr. Billig were brought after several of his open-heart patients died. He was convicted in the deaths of three of them. Witnesses said Dr. Billig was nearly blind in one eye and had made serious errors.

In his summation, Col. Gerald L. Miller, the chief prosecutor, noted that before joining the Navy Dr. Billig had been dismissed from one surgical job and had been stripped of surgical privileges at another hospital. But, Colonel Miller said, he was able to get a new surgical post after each dismissal. The only way to protect the public from Dr. Billig, he argued, would be to jail him.

The 20-page decision of the appeals court, dated Wednesday and released today, was signed by four judges and concurred in with limited reservations by three others.

Navy undecided on appeal

A Navy spokesman said that Dr. Billig was released from a barracks at Fort Leavenworth, Kan., today and will live in a bachelor officer's quarters until the end of a 20-day period for further motions. The Navy said it has not decided whether to appeal.

The court's decision will not allow Dr. Billig to resume his surgical career in the Navy, a military spokesman said. Dr. Billig's surgical and medical privileges were stripped from him in an administrative procedure, and that action is not affected by the dismissal of criminal charges.

The Navy had informed state licensing boards that Dr. Billig had been stripped of his privileges. Now, the spokesman said, the Navy will inform the civilian licensing authorities that his conviction was overturned.

The appeals court reviewed the evidence concerning the three most serious crimes for which Dr. Billig was convicted—two involuntary manslaughters and a negligent homicide—and essentially reached the opposite conclusion based on the same facts.

In a case in which death was attributed to Dr. Billig's actions, the appeals court said that the death might have been caused instead by a high level of potassium in the patient and that, at any rate, another doctor was the primary surgeon.

The court also reversed Dr. Billig's conviction on 18 counts of dereliction of duty for violating restrictions that supposedly required him to perform complicated operations under supervision for much of 1983. The court said his status was "so confused and frequently shifting" that he could not reasonably understand the restrictions.

The court said that, while Dr. Billig had bad vision in one eye, there was conflicting testimony on the degree of impairment. The court noted that he had performed 72 consecutive open-heart surgeries requiring intricate sewing.

The court also said it was wrong of the prosecution to highlight the deficiencies of another surgeon and then "impute criminal liability" to Dr. Billig as his supervisor.

The prosecutors lost sight of the fact that coronary-bypass surgery is inherently risky and performed on patients who are quite ill and apt to die, the court said.

Case 11

John McCabe and Blue Cross and Blue Shield of Michigan

Introductory Note: This is a case of hubris in health care management. McCabe's impatience led him to challenge the appointment of a controversial public board member. His arrogance in turn led to a new Blue Cross and Blue Shield (BCBSM) enabling act, which McCabe fought for several years in the courts and lost. The momentum of this action led to the diversification and mutualization campaigns. All of this served to avoid an intensive dialogue and disciplined examination of the central management question, What is the best way to preserve and improve on the success of BCBSM?

What forces exist to keep a chief executive officer (CEO) appropriately humble? One is the governing board. Others are forces more or less independent of the CEO's authority, forces like financiers, buyers, suppliers, or the hospital medical staff. Another is the executive's own personal character. None of these worked in this situation, although the players were among the most sophisticated in the country. Finally, someone discovered problems with a condominium in Florida, and McCabe resigned. How could more positive forces have been made to work? What sorts of policies, corporate cultures, or procedures would have led to a stabilization and recovery at various points along the way?

Blue Cross and Blue Shield of Michigan under the Leadership of John C. McCabe*

Introduction

Blue Cross and Blue Shield of Michigan were founded under special legislation in the late 1930s as prepayment plans, not-for-profit social agencies designed to bring providers and patients together in a joint program to finance health care costs. The Blue Cross movement had great success and by the late 1970s provided almost half the private health insurance in the United States. Michigan, led in many ways by the labor-management negotiations of the United Auto Workers (UAW) and the Big Three automotive manufacturers, paralleled the national trends. By 1977, the two plans had merged and were writing broad health care benefits for nearly 5,000,000 lives. They also served as the intermediary for Medicare in Michigan and underwrote virtually all the Medicare Supplementary Insurance.

However, it was clear that the road ahead was not to be easy. There were important misgivings about the cost of health care, its impact on the competitive position of the Big Three and other Michigan companies, the broad first-dollar benefits in the most common contracts, and the lack of progress toward newer forms of health insurance that emphasized patient incentives such as deductibles and copayments and provider incentives such as managed care. Some thought it would be impossible to incorporate the kinds of changes necessary to protect BCBSM's market share; history, size, and structure would be an insuperable liability. Others thought that the job could be done but that BCBSM was not moving fast enough; it needed public regulation to make it move more rapidly.

John C. McCabe, who became president of BCBSM after many years of experience and a term as president of Blue Shield before its merger with Blue Cross in 1975, disagreed with both groups. He thought BCBSM could and would do the job, if it was given the freedom

---

*Summarized from reports in *The Detroit News*, 1977 to 1988, by Patricia A. Nef, with supplementary materials from court and insurance commissioner records. Excerpts from *The Detroit News* are reprinted with the permission of *The Detroit News*, a Gannett newspaper, copyright 1977 through 1988.

from regulation and liberty to act that major commercial insurance competitors had.

1977

On 22 July, Charles Chomet, project director for Citizens for Better Care Institute, who "thrived on controversy,"[1] was ousted from the board of directors. State Insurance Commissioner Tom Jones criticized BCBSM for not paying attention to public concerns; he called the removal of Chomet "'vindictive retaliation for speaking out in public and not in the board room.' "[2] The state sued for reinstatement, and a court order reappointed Chomet to the board, to which BCBSM's attorney George E. Bushnell responded that they "could 'live with Chomet' whom he called an 'irritant.' "[3] On 17 December, State Representative Perry Bullard reported the introduction of new legislation to restructure BCBSM to increase public accountability of its board and to implement cost-containment measures. "'The recent incredible arrogance of the Blue Cross-Blue Shield board in rejecting the nomination of Charles Chomet dramatizes the need for this change'," said Representative Bullard, who introduced the bill.[4]

1978

Five board members (one of them Chomet) publicly challenged the board's decision to increase McCabe's salary. The raise of $11,000 brought McCabe's salary to $121,000.

1979

On March 8, McCabe's salary increase of $9,000, bringing his yearly salary to $130,000, was approved. His salary had increased 94 percent since he started at BCBSM in 1974. A joint statement issued by UAW Vice-President Kenneth Bannon; Arthur Hughes, chairman of the labor component of the BCBSM board and a UAW representative; Robert Walker of the UAW; and Robert Brenner, an official with the Allied Industrial Workers Union called the increase "'unwarranted,' " "'excessive,' " and "'against the interests of consumers.' "[5]

1980

On 12 March, the *Detroit News* reported that Charles Chomet had been nominated for another term on the BCBSM board.

114   Improving Virtue

In late August, a version of the bill to restructure BCBSM introduced by Representative Bullard in 1977 reached the floor of the Michigan House and passed. A different version, much more sympathetic to the interests of BCBSM management, passed in the Senate. Attention focused on the conference committee, which had to reach agreement by the end of the year or both bills would die. The House provisions included

1. a restatement of the original enabling acts of BCBSM, emphasizing that it must be publicly responsible for the control of health care costs and for making access to insurance and health care available to any citizen of the state;
2. a mandate to reduce the number of governing board members from 47 to 35, to increase consumer representatives (as opposed to health care providers) from 57 percent to 74 percent, and to increase the number of these who are publicly appointed from 2 to 4;
3. assignment to the state insurance commissioner of the authority to review rates and to disapprove them if they exceed the level implied by inflation and the rate of growth of the economy; and
4. a section requiring the insurance commissioner to directly regulate rates of payment to providers and BCBSM premiums if premiums cannot be contained within these levels.

On 14 September, the *Detroit News* reported that, derived from information supplied by company officials, BCBSM was spending millions of dollars (and tens of thousands of hours of staff time) on lobbying efforts against the restructuring bill, including a $2-million-a-year statewide advertising campaign aimed at gaining public sympathy. It also noted that the lobby resulted in the Senate adopting a "Blues-written substitute" for the House bill.[6] The lobbying effort would culminate in activities designed to influence the conference committee, and the article noted, "Most of the forces opposing the Blues feel the company's efforts have nearly succeeded."[7]

Company spokesman Dennis Larson said, "'This is the major challenge in the company's 41-year history.'"[8] Lobbying efforts were described by the *News* as consisting of "a small army of Blues executives and hired experts."[9] They reported that efforts included

1. the $2 million advertising campaign;

2. a 10-member task force to research and assess legislative efforts;
3. staff members present at all hearings;
4. attempts to gain UAW legislative support by offering loans to Chrysler (Representative Hollister commented that " '[t]he loan didn't buy off the UAW... but it made it hard for the UAW to oppose Blues management. It softened them' "[10]); and
5. other attempts at gaining the faith of the community including financing aid to Detroit Receiving Hospital (the *News* said, "The investments weren't directly tied to the legislative battle, but they did buy goodwill"[11]) and increasing deposits in certain banks BCBSM used ("The Blues won friends in Michigan's banking community"[12]).

By November, the structuring bill cleared for passage as PA 350, despite the BCBSM attempts at stopping legislation. The governor signed it, to take effect on 3 April, 1981. BCBSM sought an injunction.

BCBSM's request for an injunction was granted before PA 350 could take effect. The company began a suit in circuit court to have the law declared unconstitutional. At the request of the governor, the Michigan Supreme Court ordered the circuit court to "certify the controlling questions of public law, to provide a statement of relevant facts and to conduct evidentiary hearings relative to the case."[13]

1982

Hearings were held from 27 July to 24 September, generating 4,000 pages of transcript and 194 exhibits. The circuit court filed its findings 1 November. Nine questions were identified.[14] These can be informally summarized to three:

1. Does the act unfairly invade BCBSM's operations, through the regulation of products and prices not imposed on its competition?
2. Are the provisions of the act specific enough to avoid arbitrary and capricious decisions by the insurance commissioner?
3. Does the constitution permit the legislation to mandate the governing board and other operational matters of BCBSM?

116   *Improving Virtue*

1983

On 14 September, the BCBSM board passed a measure to start a lobbying effort to make it a commercial insurance company (mutualization effort). The vote, according to McCabe, was "'substantially in favor but not unanimous.'"[15]

The company reported that market share has fallen to 49 percent, that losses for 1977 to 1982 totalled $172 million, and that 800 BCBSM jobs had been eliminated.

McCabe commented that changing to a mutual would "help stop 'the erosion of our market share and our membership losses by placing us for the first time on an equal footing with our out-of-state commercial competitors.'"[16]

The *Detroit News* reported that BCBSM "had complained for years that state insurance commissioners applied tough and unfair regulatory actions against the Blues while doing little to regulate the other 340 licensed commercial carriers."[17] BCBSM succeeded in getting UAW support for the movement; UAW vice-president Donald Ephlin worked on the proposal and commented in the *News* that "'the company is losing a contest being waged on an uneven field.'"[18]

A letter to the editor of the *Detroit News* from Attorney General Frank Kelley stated that BCBSM's market share was increasing, not decreasing: "in 1980 the Blues collected over $2.3 billion in premiums, or 61.54 percent of the total health-care premiums collected in Michigan.... in 1982, the Blues market share was over 69 percent...."[19] He noted that the two leading out-of-state competitors had a combined market share of less than 5 percent. He claimed that BCBSM was "unhappy because the umpire, as it were, ruled against them [in their requests for rate increases] and unable to appeal to change the umpire's decision, the Blues instead want to change the rules of the game.... They think government should simply give them benefits like a tax-free status, and ask no questions...."[20]

On 9 October, the *Detroit News* reported that BCBSM was already "somewhat diversified."[21] On the nonprofit side there were two subsidiaries that coordinated its HMOs and operated a research foundation (Health Services Co.). On the for-profit side, it had a computer services company (Diversitec) and a company that packaged insurance (Blue Ribbon Inc.). McCabe said that, should BCBSM become commercial, there would be more extensive diversification. He also noted that one of the possibilities was a medical credit card system. In addition, he said, "having some direct role in the provision of care, through joint ventures or related efforts" was a potentially long-range plan.[22] Regarding the mutualization effort, McCabe said that, should the conversion not be allowed, BCBSM did not have another option ready. "'We haven't given up on "Plan A" yet. . . . It may take a little longer than we expected. . . . We really don't have a "Plan B." We'll have a "Plan B" when we're sure "Plan A" won't work.'"[23] McCabe also commented that there might be increased opposition to the mutualization effort due to the 1983 financial results but that those in opposition would be "people who don't 'understand a balance sheet.'"[24]

The attorney general's office and BCBSM disagreed on most of the facts surrounding the issue. Harry Iwasko, from the state attorney's office, said, "'If they kept losing money like they claim, they'd be bankrupt.'"[25]

1984

Lawsuits filed by the attorney general and the insurance commissioner contended that BCBSM was illegally involved in the development and use of two subsidiaries in the Caribbean. BCBSM officials claimed to be "merely taking steps to meet the needs and demands of consumers and to assure that their company succeeds," according to the *Detroit News*.[26] The insurance commissioner called the strategy a "'national shell game' created to 'avoid regulation and circumvent the law'" and the attorney general was quoted as saying, "'It's a rip-off.'"[27] McCabe (a "$228,572-a-year president and chief executive"[28]) and other BCBSM executives held almost all the decision-making positions of the subsidiaries. The BCBSM statement justifying its use of subsidiaries stated that it was "'facing limited growth and intensifying competition in its basic business of prepaid health care coverage. The formula for longterm survival includes the flexibility to develop new products to meet changing customer needs and to diversify to support our core business.'"[29]

Three major focuses became apparent in the diversification plan. The first was the Caribbean plan. The attorney general's lawsuit alleged that BCBSM was "'believed to be funnelling money out of the country. . .where its use is not subject to the review of the commissioner of insurance.'"[30] The plan was thought to work as follows: health coverage was transferred to the Chicago BCS Insurance Co. (owned by the national Blue Cross and Blue Shield Association); BCS ceded the Michigan business to Central Insurance Ltd. (in the Cayman Islands) or to Business Group Insurance Ltd. (in Nassau, the Bahamas); these two companies were subsidiaries of BCBSM's Health Service Co. and Blue Ribbon Inc.

Blue Cross and Blue Shield's justification was that its subsidiaries had set up these foreign subsidiaries to "'provide BCBSM and its HMOs with low cost reinsurance for stop-loss and other liability insurance not otherwise available at reasonable rates.'"[31] State officials thought otherwise. They believed the use of foreign subsidiaries was to avoid regulation and taxes. They were unable to accurately determine the size of the operation because they were denied access to the books. (The subsidiaries were considered separate legal entities from BCBSM over which the state had no authority.)

The second subject of investigation was the use of wholly owned subsidiary Blue Ribbon Inc. to sell life insurance. BCBSM, which operated under a unique statute of charter, P.A. 108 and 109, was not permitted by its charter to sell such insurance. BCBSM stated that there was "'nothing unusual about such arrangements.'"[32] The third was a diversification activity that allowed BCBSM to offer billing systems to doctors at less than competitive rates through the use of subsidiary Diversitec.

A report issued by company auditors noted "a 'lack of control over the entire real estate operation.'"[33]

1985

On 17 April, P.A. 350 was upheld by a four-to-one vote in the Michigan Supreme Court. The opinion went almost entirely against BCBSM, reversing only a few of the operational "invasions." The finding emphasized the public duties historically imposed on BCBSM and noted among other things that the court had noted in 1978 that the insurance commissioner lacked power to regulate health care costs and had "filled the gap by construing the enabling legislation broadly."[34] The Court remarked that "The Legislature responded quickly... [with] 1980 PA 350...."[35] Throughout the opinion, the court dismissed BCBSM claims, describing them as "unsubstantial," "misplaced," and in one instance, "overblown and unsubstantiated as compared with what the statute actually provides."[36]

Shortly after the court decision, the attorney general sought permission to investigate BCBSM finances. Assistant Attorney General Harry Iwasko called BCBSM financial statements "'outlandish.... They are not impossible but certainly improbable.'"[37] A BCBSM spokesperson said the high reserve for unpaid claims was only temporary, due to delayed submissions of claims.

On 4 May, McCabe claimed that the court decision to uphold the 1980 law would "'destroy'" BCBSM.[38] He said that BCBSM would seek legislative approval to become a mutual insurance company, thus giving up its tax-free status. McCabe commented, "'I'm not willing to lie down and die.... We are a big organization and I will try like hell to keep it that way.'"[39] Attorney General Kelley commented that BCBSM had an "'arrogant attitude toward the public interest.'"[40] A BCBSM spokesperson responded, "'We are shocked by the attorney general's invective and his personal attack and we have no intention of responding in kind.'"[41]

On 1 June, the *Detroit News* reported that BCBSM accused Kelley of being "'hell-bent on crippling Blue Cross and Blue Shield by harassment and abusive state regulation.'"[42] The week earlier, Kelley had announced plans to implement a media campaign against the BCBSM mutualization attempt. In response to the BCBSM reaction to the request to review their books, Kelley stated, "'Their irrational reaction should cause all reasonable people to wonder what they have to hide.'"[43]

On 24 June, a stay for the implementation of P.A. 350 pending appeal to the U.S. Supreme Court was denied along with a motion for a rehearing, and implementation of the law began. On 28 July, the *Detroit News* reported that McCabe blamed financial losses on the "'hostile regulatory climate.'"[44] The attorney general's office responded, "'Mismanagement maybe, but not overregulation.'"[45]

On 7 October, the U.S. Supreme Court rejected an appeal to hear the BCBSM case. The *Detroit News* reported that "[t]he Blues will seek legislation to negate the 1980 law by becoming a nonprofit mutual insurance company...."[46]

On 10 October, the *Detroit News* reported that Kelley attacked the BCBSM mutualization effort, "calling its management 'greedy,' its advertising 'lies' and their statements 'distortions.'"[47] Both sides accused the other of misstatements of fact.

On 28 December, the *Detroit News* reported that Kelley was charging BCBSM with not properly complying with the now-implemented 1980 law. He claimed that BCBSM "deliberately [drafted] new bylaws the insurer knew would not be approved by the state—thus delaying implementation of the law even further."[48] In a letter to McCabe, Kelley wrote, "'The action by the company in this matter appears most irresponsible.'"[49] In the letter, the *News* reported that Kelley also "chided

Blues officials for attempting to 'silence criticism' and 'orchestrate' the outcome of the board selection process. . . ."[50] BCBSM officials claimed to have not yet seen the letter. Vice-President for Corporate Communications Dick Femmel commented, "'To suggest [the board members] are pawns of current management is ludicrous.'"[51]

1986

On 26 January, the *Detroit News* reported that after spending over $1.5 million on advertising and promotion for their mutualization effort, BCBSM appeared to have lost the battle. Sources within BCBSM said possible reasons for the failure included McCabe's disregard of advice that an election year was not a good year to introduce controversial legislation, the criticisms of the bill by Governor Blanchard's legal advisor, and the failure of BCBSM to gain the support of the UAW and senior citizens groups.

1987

In late October, the BCBSM board initiated an investigation of the purchase of a condominium in Florida by a BCBSM subsidiary, to be conducted by the audit committee. As reported in the *Detroit News*, 29 October 1987, in question was the purchase of a townhouse in the exclusive Professional Golf Association (PGA) National Golf Course resort area by BCBSM subsidiary H.C. Real Estate Co. McCabe owned a condo in the same area and allegedly wished to upgrade. The condo was in a "'non-premium area'" and the market for its resale might have been limited.[52] The PGA agreed to buy back the condo for $1,000 more than was paid for it on the condition that H.C. Real Estate purchase a $183,000 townhome in the PGA area. McCabe was thus able to easily sell his condo as well as to avoid transaction fees. While the PGA lost money on the resale of McCabe's condo, the loss was made up in the purchase of the H.C. Real Estate Co. townhome. The deal was allegedly worked out by McCabe.

The state's attorney general office, along with the insurance commissioners office, began their own investigation. The investigations included additional areas of misuse of funds, including the installation of security systems in the homes of BCBSM executives; house, lawn, and pool repairs provided by H.C. Real Estate Co.; the employment of relatives of top managers; various country club memberships; and the purchase of company cars by executives, who then sold the cars under value to associates and friends (three executives bought 29 cars between them since 1980).

In early December, McCabe was asked to step down as chairman and CEO. A board audit committee report stated that McCabe "'violated the spirit and the intent'" of the law.[53]

On 9 December, the *Detroit News* reported that one board member partially blamed the misuse of funds on the freedom and lack of controls brought by one person's being chairman of the board and CEO at the same time. That director said that in the future the board would have to decide "'whether the chief executive officer ever will be chairman again. There's a significant portion of the board that believes that is not a good idea to allow power to be consolidated, control of the board and the agenda being in managements' hands.'"[54] That member also stated that if the *News* hadn't reported the misuse of funds, "two thirds of the members of the board wouldn't have had any idea of any of them.'"[55]

1988

The *Detroit News* reported on 9 January that BCBSM interim chairman, Richard E. Whitmer, and the BCBSM board were reviewing its "corporate philosophy."[56] Included in this review was the proposal to drop McCabe's idea of converting to a private, mutual insurance company. In the examination of BCBSM subsidiaries, Whitmer said, according to the News, "it is his hope that any subsidiaries surviving the review, [sic] would have boards of directors and chairmen who are from outside Blue Cross."[57] Whitmer also emphasized establishing a better relationship with BCBSM regulators.

On 4 March, the *News* reported that a state audit had announced that BCBSM was in poor financial condition and should "consider restructuring or dumping" various subsidiaries.[58] According to the *News*, the BCBSM directors were told by the state audit that "[l]osses resulted from gross management blunders."[59] On 6 March, the *News* reported that the audit showed BCBSM had "pumped nearly $120 million into 20 subsidiary companies during the last nine years, but [had] gotten little return on its investment."[60]

On 9 April, the *Detroit News* reported that BCBSM had lost a record $331 million in 1987.

Table IV.1 and Figures IV.2–IV.4 summarize the financial performance of BCBSM, and Table IV.2 shows McCabe's compensation.

122 *Improving Virtue*

Table IV.1 Blue Cross and Blue Shield of Michigan Financial Performance, 1980–1988 (millions of dollars)

Year	Premiums Earned	Underwriting Gain (Loss)	Net Gain (Loss)	Reserves in Dollars
1980	$2,355	($ 99.47)	($ 34.72)	$236
1981	2,640	(96.30)	(54.50)	180
1982	2,921	(12.09)	34.76	216
1983	3,100	49.34	108.55	322
1984	3,285	(8.00)	45.18	359
1985	3,344	(15.81)	20.41	379
1986	3,906	(41.68)	(6.98)	369
1987	3,967	(244.04)	(223.02)	95
1988	4,284	(114.22)	(79.34)	29

Source: Annual reports to the Michigan Insurance Bureau.

Table IV.2 John C. McCabe's Compensation, 1977–1988

Year	Salary	Increase
1977	$110,000	94% since 1974
1978	121,000	10%
1979	130,000	7%
1984	228,572	76% since 1979
1986	388,041	70% since 1984
1987	400,000	negligible
1988	662,974	(includes accumulated leave)

Source: Reports in the *Detroit News*.

Figure IV.2 Blue Cross and Blue Shield of Michigan Premiums Earned by Year, 1980–1988

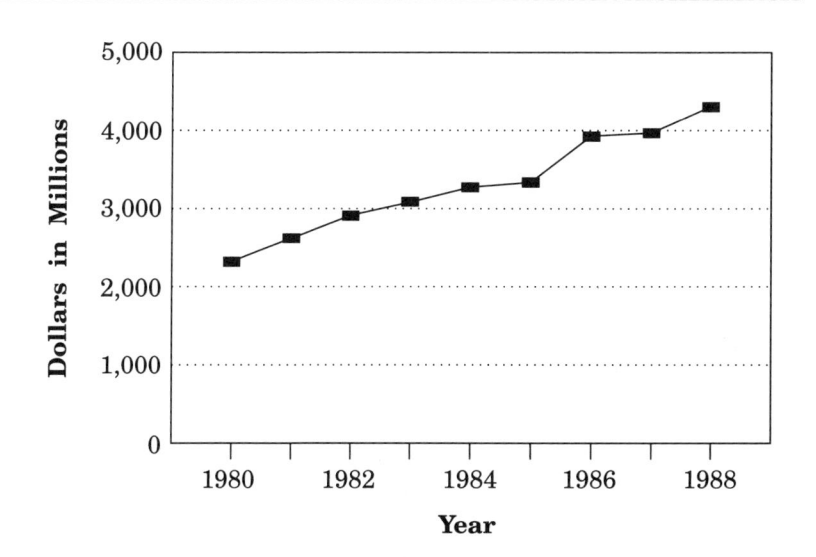

Figure IV.3 Blue Cross and Blue Shield of Michigan Net Gain by Year, 1980–1988

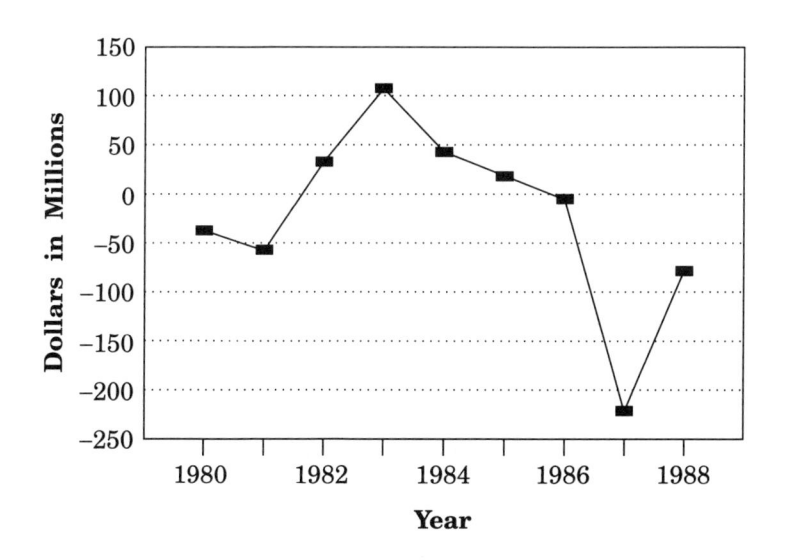

Figure IV.4 Blue Cross and Blue Shield of Michigan Days of Reserve by Year, 1980–1988

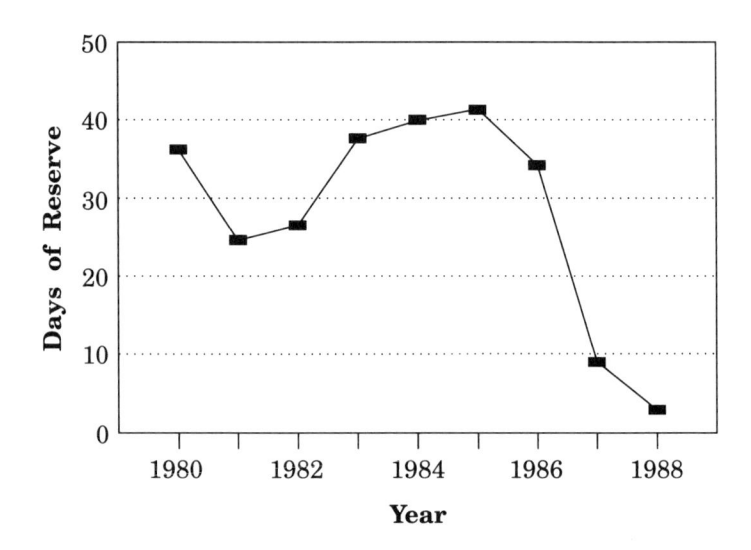

Part IV Commentary

Building the Virtuous Health Care Corporation

The Concept of Moral Virtue

The moral challenge of health care management clearly takes several forms. Occasionally it can involve disputes over the moral limits of the enterprise, as in the abortion and neonatal rights cases. Frequently it involves the weighing of *prima facie* obligations, the often contradictory dictates of beneficence and justice. Perpetually it returns to the question of the moral failure of bureaucratic organizations and their leaders. Can evil be made less banal? Are hubris and corruption the inevitable consequences of power? Can managers and workers improve their individual moral performances, and if so, can organizations help them? The central purpose of bureaucratic organizations is "to help common people do uncommon things."[61] Modern health care has done surprisingly well with this objective in a nonmoral context; can we also use health care organizations to help people to uncommon moral achievements?

A few definitions and clarifications are useful in considering the question of moral virtue in either a personal or an organizational context. The theories of moral obligation suggest that a virtuous person is one who does the right thing, but important caveats are necessary to take into account intention, freedom, and ability. Moral virtue is generally taken to include intention. Sacrifice in a futile effort to do the right act is virtuous; the right act undertaken by accident is not. Freedom is clearly important; an individual who could not have affected the situation does not lose virtue by not acting. The question of ability is less clear. It can be looked on as identical to freedom; an individual is only free to do what is within his or her abilities. But one of the real contributions of bureaucratic organizations is their power to extend limits and expand ability. To conclude that virtue consists only of good intentions and good actions within some limit of ability to act is superficial because good management can expand the limit. Thus the goal of moral management is to improve moral virtue in three ways:

1. Increase the *intentions* of managers and other individuals in organizations to perform right acts.
2. Increase the *freedom* to perform right acts.
3. Increase the *ability* to perform right acts.

We will pursue these goals by reviewing the cases briefly and then examining four topics: the personal promotion of moral virtue, the justification for leadership and command, the role of reward and retribution in promoting moral virtue, and a summary of the opportunities for leaders to promote moral virtue in organizations.

Can Nonmoral Actions Promote Moral Virtue? A Review of the Cases

Perhaps the first step to moral virtue is humility, recognizing that "there but for the grace of God go I." The things that distinguish the individuals and the institutions whose virtue fails them are likely to be much smaller than we would like to think. The second, as usual, is the careful review of nonmoral systems.

Moral virtue begins with resistance to temptation, the expedient material benefit actually or illusorily available at the expense of making someone else the means. The first case simply identifies some common temptations, both obvious and subtle. The various temptations to be resisted show that ethical behavior depends mainly on individual will, but the role of an organizational response soon becomes apparent. Good policies promote strong wills.

The first element of will is a clear understanding of the moral issues involved, that is, why a certain answer is morally preferred. Extensions of the principles of beneficence and justice to a professional work commitment make the virtuous responses clear. If patients, health care purchasers, and other employees are not to be used as means, gifts that threaten equity must be declined. Actions that endanger the organization's needs are to be avoided, including those that endanger your own health. Ethical codes, such as those at the end of Part I, clarify and support such a professional commitment.

Some apparent *prima facie* conflicts arise, but many do not survive critical review. "The board doesn't object to this," "My boss told me it was okay," and "Everybody does it," of course do not make it right; rather they suggest the need for a deliberate strategy. When these attitudes exist, they reflect failures in the corporate culture that can be difficult to change. Virtue does not call for a pompous public display. It calls for a thoughtful and effective effort to correct the problem.

Even at a relatively simple level, formal organizational policies that reinforce the correct response are desirable. They reassure the uncertain, they overwhelm the rationalizations, and they point the direction for the harder questions. Similarly, example seems to be powerful. While people might not copy a virtuous leader, they are quick to use the failings of a more human one to justify their own temptations.

The Bethesda Naval Hospital, St. Elizabeth's, and BCBSM cases are tragedies of a higher order. Lives were lost or severely damaged; careers were ruined; health insurance for four million people was endangered. Three prominent, otherwise respected organizations were publicly condemned. Members and patients of these institutions who had nothing to do with the events cited suffered along with those directly involved. How can horrors like these be prevented?

The individual doctors Burt and Billig have one set of moral problems; the organizations that privileged them have another. Under both legal and moral extensions of beneficence and justice, a hospital is obligated to obtain data and to take steps to ensure that the quality of performance of its staff is adequate.[62] Otherwise it exploits a position of trust given by the community. Christ's or Maimonides's tests of justice, that you or your loved one would undergo surgery from the doctors you privileged, are excruciating here. Why then did no one act?

The privileging and credentialing systems of hospitals are supposed to prevent occurrences like these. Furthermore, The Joint Commission on Accreditation of Healthcare Organizations (JCAHO) exists to make sure that hospitals uphold their privileging obligations. Both of these organizations have held JCAHO accreditation throughout the 1980s.[63] The two hospitals and the JCAHO strive for virtue when they conduct their privileges review. In these cases, they failed to stop these two surgeons from doing harm. (The fact that the processes failed suggests they can be improved but not necessarily that they should be replaced. One would replace the processes if one had evidence that a replacement would be more effective.)

The reasons why nothing was done include the weighing of *prima facie* obligations. Captain Hodges testified Commodore Quinn pressured him to put the existence of a cardiovascular surgery program ahead of the danger to the patients. He appears to have put his duty to accept a military order ahead of his duty to attend the privileging hearing, a complicated question for a career officer.

At St. Elizabeth's, many questions were raised, but few before the late 1970s. *American Medical News* reported that several nurses complained in 1973 about Dr. Burt's excessive use of obstetric anesthesia. (Deep anesthesia would be necessary to undertake the extensive reconstructions, but it threatens the newborn.) One nurse reported she was told, "'As long he's not killing patients, we have to put up with him,'" by the then director of nursing.[64] She apparently resigned as a result of that response. Another nurse reported that the hospital administrator, now deceased, told her in 1974 that "'I can't get one doctor to stand up and say that what Burt does is out of the current realm of medical practice.'"[65] According to the *Dayton Daily News*, the surgical tissue committee questioned Dr. Burt's surgical judgment in two cases unrelated to the "love surgery" in 1977, and he was given a conditional reappointment. In late 1978 the medical executive committee asked him to document the benefits of the "love surgery" and began insisting on special, more complete documentation of patients' informed consents.[66] According to *American Medical News*, Dr. Burt responded with an extensive report including a "before and after survey of his surgery's impact."[67] The survey was sent to "more than 200 former patients; 55 responded, and the answers to the vast majority of questions were resoundingly positive."[68]

Apparently on the basis of that evidence, the executive committee decided that Dr. Burt could continue the surgery using the more rigorous consent form. In 1979, additional questions were raised about his surgical judgement.[69] In addition, some doctors seem to have tried to get help earlier from the Ohio State Board of Medicine, but their requests were not answered. As Dr. Hilty notes, fear of legal retribution might be another reason the Dayton medical community was not more aggressive. "'Legal counsel for the hospital thought there was a potential [antitrust] liability if they took further action,'" one doctor said.[70]

Thus the problem lingered. Despite the concerns of many people, it was never definitively addressed. Virtue calls for any of them—it might have taken only one in each case—to have taken action, but action was virtuous, not obligatory. In each case, the individuals faced substantial risks of retribution, and they were not obliged to place themselves or their families at risk.

Similar conflicts between obligations to self, the organization, and the customer are only to be expected in serious situations like the St. Elizabeth's and Bethesda cases. The management requirement is for an environment where problems are detected and objectively reviewed, as promptly as possible. The technical keys to that environment are well-designed procedures; good data systems; and routine, objective reviews of performance. The corporate culture keys are carefully selected leaders who will encourage both prompt investigation and objective review, deliberate protection of the innocent and those who might be falsely accused, and sufficient diversity of participation to minimize the exposure of any one person.

The perceived threat of lawsuits in the Burt case might be the critical factor. Any doctor unreasonably denied privileges may sue. He or she is entitled to due process. Even if he or she fails in the suit, there are problems of public exposure and cost for the whistleblowers once the suit is placed. But the hospital can protect the doctors on the review committee. Clear criteria, comprehensive data, candid discussion, and explicit policies about the review process would certainly help medical staff members reach a more virtuous decision.[71] Procedurally, the organization can either encourage or discourage these elements of privileges review. Data come from well-maintained medical records. Criteria are developed over time, by capable medical leadership. A committee secretary taking accurate minutes and familiar with relevant bylaws is important. A deliberate separation of the privileging process from other goals of operations, such as the retention of a specific program or the income of specific physicians, helps. A tradition that the patient should come first would certainly be in the right direction. A tradition of confidentiality and an understanding that the identification of a problem is not the same as an accusation of moral failure would have allowed both institutions to reach the right decisions and save lives years earlier.

The McCabe case is more difficult. It is the board's role to restrain the CEO, but there are no perfect governance models. Being CEO of a multibillion-dollar corporation takes a lot of ego strength; it is not surprising either that some CEOs are consumed by the same talents that got them to the top or that governing boards occasionally fail. One could write a few new bylaws, but there is no guarantee that they would work. The board nominating committee should have more independence, the audit committee should come in sooner, and the board chair should be someone who represents the customers of BCBSM rather than the CEO. At a somewhat more helpful level, the board compensation committee should emphasize the buyers' and members' perspectives. While the level of McCabe's compensation might be justified, the steady increase in the face of deteriorating performance is highly questionable.

The only real organizational protection against the kind of problem the case represents is the board's vigorous, objective review of performance each year. This is the *environmental assessment* required to start the budget process and identify the objectives for the coming year. It can also be used as a basis for compensating the CEO and other top executives. In a company the size of BCBSM, it should have the direct participation of the most critical stakeholders. (Chomet should not have been dismissed; he should have been given a voice among others in preparing the environmental assessment.) The effective board has to be composed only of those who are willing to work for the organization's success, because they must seriously commit themselves to hard, disciplined work. This requirement suggests either a smaller board or an executive committee with limited terms and frequent reelection by the stakeholders.

In the end, all the cases come down to moral leadership. A few people willing to speak candidly and to act are often enough to turn the tide. If some of the individuals who played key roles had acted in different ways, the cases would never have existed. What then can be done to encourage the virtuous response in yourself and in other members of your organization?

Why Lead a Moral Life?
The Personal Promotion of Moral Virtue

One of the interesting characteristics of modern professional life is the relationship of material reward and moral virtue. Managers, doctors, lawyers, soldiers, and engineers can easily enhance their material rewards by curtailing moral virtue. Not only are promotions, higher fees, bonuses, and stock options based on nonmoral achievement, they are frequently easier to achieve if one is not too scrupulous. Only rarely does society stop to reward moral virtue, and when it does, either the case is extreme or the individual has died. Possibly as a result, the world is plagued with insider stock trading, unnecessary surgery, frivolous lawsuits, hidden dumps of contaminated waste, and rockets with faulty seals.

In not-for-profit and governmental health care organizations, the material temptations to moral equivocation might be less, but public recognition of moral virtue is no more common. Moral virtue is expected, not rewarded. The individuals in the cases were unlikely to have received prizes for *not* doing the things they did. The Navy would not have given Dr. Quinn a medal for stopping Dr. Billig and interrupting the heart surgery program. Had someone at St. Elizabeth's blown the whistle on Dr. Burt, he or she could quite likely have been penalized. John McCabe would not have been more handsomely compensated; there was no prize for patience, humility, or tolerance of the views of others.

The first problem, therefore, is to develop incentives for moral virtue. It appears these must come initially from within the individual, at least at the leadership level. There must be an intrinsic sense of reward, even of joy, at achieving the right act. The fulfillment of obligations must be its own reward. At the same time, there must be a counterbalancing sense of humility, of willingness to hear contrary viewpoints. A sense of the corruption possible from power and a willingness to limit oneself are essential.

It is not clear where individuals acquire these characteristics. Early education, family, and religious commitment seem to be important, but there are almost as many exceptions as examples. The ability to fulfill personal needs without excess material goods is important, but we do not know how to teach that ability. We are no further along with this problem than Socrates. We know only that individuals differ in moral capacity and that in some vague way, examining one's objectives, life, and beliefs is important to developing capacity for virtue.

However, those who have examined their lives and those who have demonstrated moral capacity in the past do appear to be better candidates for future moral virtue. Perhaps the best avenues to promote moral virtues among health care leaders are selection and self-selection. Selection has two elements, direct and indirect. Directly, those who have given evidence of moral virtue should be preferred over those who have not. Indirectly, by promoting health care as an avenue to satisfaction through service, rather than through wealth, power, or worldly adulation, we can discourage entry by those whose greed and ambition would fit a more aggressive environment. Those who have difficulty with the limits of the field can be encouraged to find some other career where material rewards are higher but where environmental forces protect society from excesses. These considerations suggest that we should always encourage moral virtue as part of our selection and promotion policies, including those for admission to professional education. Our stance should reflect the reality:

there is only modest material reward here and great opportunity for moral satisfaction.

To make this strategy practical, we must improve the relative importance of intrinsic rewards for moral virtue and advertise what these are. Clearly such rewards exist. Most of us would agree with Socrates that, "The unexamined life is not worth living."[72] Intrinsic rewards lie in gratification from the achievements themselves: the healing of the sick, the relief of pain and suffering, the fulfillment of personal objectives, the satisfaction of contribution to the common good, and the joy of working with like-minded colleagues. The cynic will say that intrinsic rewards are meaningless, that nice guys finish last. Yet the evidence is stronger to the contrary: nice guys have lives of material comfort and enjoy the deeper satisfaction of contributing to the moral good. It is in fact the material rewards that are meaningless, in the sense that they never replace these gratifications. There is a legion of anecdote, a mythology, that supports the power of intrinsic rewards. The foundation of programs to enhance virtue must begin by endorsing and fostering this reward.

The long and the short of it is we have no reward greater than that of a job well done. There is, in the end, no improvement on Socrates' "Apology." "A man who is good for anything ought not to calculate the chance of living or dying, he ought only to consider whether in doing anything he is doing right or wrong—acting the part of the good man or the bad."[73] Or as restated only a century ago, "The only reward of virtue is virtue; the only way to have a friend is to be one."[74] Then the only way to have a virtuous organization is to be a virtuous manager and to encourage subordinates to be virtuous, by all the tools we can discover. We must make the morally well-done job easier to achieve and make it more obvious when it has occurred.

When Is Command Moral?

Obviously, one of the tools managers have to promote moral virtue is the hierarchy of communication that defines the organization. But this raises two questions relating to how to use the hierarchy and its tradition of superiority most effectively. The first question is our moral right to command: What is the moral justification of the conventional authority of superior over subordinate? The second is in the nature and use of blame: When is it appropriate to punish or to blame a subordinate?

The moral justification for authority

At bottom, several of the cases in this part and the discussion of *prima facie* obligations in Part III are related to the issue of when and how one person should assume authority over another. The question has two parts: When is there a right to command, and when is there an obligation to command?

To a certain extent, any employment contract can be viewed as a potential departure from the Kantian ideal. The bureaucratic organization has an inherent risk that the employee will become a means to an end. Authority, the right to command, itself represents a conflict between *prima facie* obligations to the employee and to the organization. However, there are two important moral justifications for authority. These are the greater good of society as a whole and the voluntary acceptance of the subordinate, to fulfill his or her own ends.[75]

The wording itself—*greater good, acceptance*—suggests that the superior holds a *prima facie* obligation not to sacrifice the subordinate to the needs of the organization, that the right to command is limited both by the acceptance of the subordinate and by the relative importance of the *prima facie* obligations to the employee and to others. While the employee's own judgment and acceptance is certainly the correct starting point, it is necessary to recognize that the employee might be under pressures to sacrifice himself or herself, and the employee's acceptance alone does not justify the management right. Under this thinking, a beneficent and just manager must limit requests of subordinates to those actions that will do no harm, either moral or nonmoral, to any party involved. It also leads to a conclusion many do not expect, that the role of the superior is to teach, to explain, to facilitate, to help, to lead, to encourage, and to ask but rarely to order.[76] An order implies an action against the employee's will. The morally preferred use of authority is to convince the employee that the action is in his or her interest.

By extension, these requirements illustrate the moral wisdom of what is already nonmorally accepted. Good management is a matter of providing information, incentive, and opportunity and of involving the subordinate in the decision processes. It is a matter of gaining the subordinate's commitment on the right thing to do, not of command at all in its customary sense. These are notions preached continuously by leaders in management thought such as Drucker,[77] Deming,[78] Juran,[79] and Mintzberg.[80]

The moral obligation of authority

The Dr. Billig and Dr. Burt cases, however, are moral failures to command when command is required, to accept the obligation of peer review and the privileging process, and to force a stop to practices that are endangering patients. These cases are dramatic but otherwise unexceptional illustrations of commonplace health care management problems. They show that command is morally required when an individual in an organization endangers others. While managers should use their authority to teach and encourage whenever the issue involves communicating what should be done, when the subordinate has demonstrated unwillingness or inability to accept the commitment to virtue, and is acting in a way that impairs the rights of others, the superior is obligated to act. Moral virtue is promoted if the action is timely, appropriate, and effective. To fail to act is to encourage the subordinate to go further and others to copy him or her. The privileges of leadership are extended by society in recognition of an acceptance of the obligation to command when necessary.

Is Punishment Wise? The Uses of Blame and Retribution in Management

Following the argument for obligation to command, the moral failure of BCBSM is not McCabe's alone. The governing board, the insurance commissioner, and the attorney general of Michigan were established to review McCabe's actions. Whether or not they did so in a timely manner raises the question of the appropriateness of blame and punishment. The same question underlies the reversal of the court martial for Dr. Billig. To what extent should we blame the individuals directly involved or those who might have been in a position to prevent the damage? And if we decide that people are blameworthy, should they be punished? The McCabe case can serve to show three issues related to this question: the cost of determining the truth, the sharing of responsibility, and the moral and nonmoral contribution of punishment.

First, the facts in the McCabe case and most complex cases are difficult to judge. The board, the commissioner, and the attorney general all acted, as did the legislature and the courts. Whether their actions were acceptably timely, appropriate, and effective or whether they should share blame with McCabe involves consideration of what others might have done under similar circumstances and a reconstruction of the intentions and ability of these parties. In the kind of complexity that this case and many health care management decisions involve, it is almost impossible to imagine what might have been. Only the most painstaking reconstruction could approach recreating the actual conditions these people worked in. (A perspective on their problem is easy to get. Place a paper over Figure IV.3 and begin moving it slowly to the right, asking yourself, Would I blow the whistle now? Or now? as more and more of the graph becomes visible.)

Second, let us suppose we could establish blame and we wanted to bear the cost of doing so. We would soon face an even tougher question: where does blame stop? Several of the board members are appointed by other agencies or jurisdictions; are these agencies also to blame? Should we blame the judicial system of Michigan, BCBSM customers (who comprise half the state population), or the electorate? When we reach this point, it becomes clear blame has no end. While there were greedy, short-sighted, inattentive, and incompetent people in the cases, to a certain extent we are all that, and to a certain extent we are all to blame. In complex matters, blame is almost always shared. Punishment of a few is scapegoating, a clear violation of Kant's rule.

There is finally the problem that determining blame might do no good, and punishment might do less. Restoration is impossible in each of three cases, and retribution might cost more than it is worth. The obligation of health care managers is not to punish the guilty but to optimize the future benefit of the system. The energies devoted to retribution do not directly improve the future; they divert resources from it. Only if retribution provides a substantial disincentive to future immorality can it be morally justified by a manager. The evidence suggests that the deterrent effect is limited and short lived. No one will emulate McCabe in Detroit or Burt in Dayton for a few years whether they are punished or not. Someone will emulate each of them sooner or later, some place or other, whether they are punished or not. While it might sometimes be necessary to blame or to punish the bad, it is often better to encourage or to reward what it right. There is more to be gained from prevention than from retribution.

Can a Manager Be a Moral Leader?

A moral manager will gain personal reward from doing what is right, from "acting the part of the good man," as Socrates put it.[81] He or she will want to promote moral virtue beyond simply doing a good job, by encouraging others to seek the same rewards. It appears that the manager has two tools to promote moral virtue among others: by example and by using the nonmoral systems of the modern organization to promote moral ends. The briefest review of history makes it clear that these mechanisms are not perfect. We cannot afford to find out whether they are effective enough to be worth the effort. It is not that moral leadership is our best hope for a better world; it is our only hope. It is the faith of our leaders that keeps our society from moral collapse. If you want to be a leader, you should accept the challenge.

Promoting moral virtue by example

It might be that the best way to promote morality in organizations is for its leaders to be both morally and nonmorally good; that strong leadership can promote morality among subordinates; and that weak leadership, whether moral or immoral, encourages morally lax responses. In terms of the theory of moral virtue, management must have the intention, the freedom, and the ability to promote moral behavior. In this context, freedom and ability relate to the resources and capability of the whole organization, as well as to the individuals. Moral leadership should begin at the top, where the greatest freedom to act exists. It is clear that nonmoral leaders build strong organizations. Moral leaders build strong organizations that have more freedom and ability to respond morally. If the leadership is strong both morally and nonmorally, it will build organizations that increase both people's intention and ability to act morally.

In a real world, it does not matter where the leader starts. Life and management are a series of moral challenges. Some will be won and some lost, and what matters is the ratio of victories to defeats. It is certainly not necessary to be perfect to be a moral leader; if it were, our plight would be dire indeed. Yesterday's sins do not preclude today's moral victories. Each event stands independent of the ones that preceded it, except for the moral growth of the individual. What is needed is to strive for perfection and to make clear that the striving is in itself rewarding. With the acceptance of the inevitability of failure, tolerance and humility become contributory virtues.

Nonmoral actions that promote moral behavior

Beyond example, are there ways to run organizations that promote morality? Can an individual in an organization help colleagues make moral decisions? I believe that the opportunity to promote moral virtue in health care organizations is much greater than it might appear. Many of the necessary steps are actually high-quality nonmoral management. None of the cases contradicts the consensus of sound theory for nonmoral management. Using that theory as a guide leads to the following conclusions:

1. Moral leadership is essential, and the higher the rank of the leader, the more important his or her moral character is. Not only should top management and governance be moral, they should be visibly moral. They must take moral stands and deliberately advertise their choices.

2. The systems and procedures of the organization should be designed to encourage the right act. Complete and accurate records, easy methods to report problems and wrongdoing, rehabilitation programs for substance abuse, internal controls on resources, safe operating environments, sound bylaws, and deliberate procedures to protect individual rights all help promote moral virtue. When they are missing, it is harder to do right.

3. Deliberate efforts should be made to build a work group that supports moral behavior and discourages immoral behavior. Expedient solutions should be discouraged. Actions that use others as means must be minimized. Destructive action must be promptly stopped. The organization must express these positions in its policies, training programs, and operational decisions. The three should be coordinated to avoid appearing hypocritical; an organization that says it puts the patient first should invest in guest relations training, have policies that are perceptive of patient needs, and maintain an environment that is safe and hospitable.

4. Workers should be empowered to the greatest extent possible, and the management style should be participative. Management should establish an environment where difficult issues can be discussed. In particular, top management should encourage debate and respect dissent, to identify the best ideas and to give tangible support to the rights of individuals. To do so requires well-designed and uniformly enforced rules of behavior. Managers should be trained in leading discussion and using consensus-building techniques to minimize the discomfort of participants. Management at all levels should be

138   Improving Virtue

prepared to respond effectively to answer any work-related question thoroughly, candidly, and as productively as possible.

5. The organization should offer moral counsel and support. The first level of support is the direct supervisor. This person should be prepared to answer moral questions as well as nonmoral ones. Given the complexity of the issues, moral counsel and support is no longer a simple matter. Ethics committees and other resources must be available to support the supervisor and the worker.

6. The organization's visible incentives, both nonmonetary and monetary, should be based on reward more than blame, but individuals threatening the moral structure or the organization's viability must be promptly removed or rehabilitated. The rewards begin with the work environment; the rules above promote an environment that makes work itself rewarding. Symbolic rewards are probably useful. Cash rewards and prizes to the worthy might not be necessary if it is clear that they do not accrue to the unworthy.

7. Standard methods of persuasion, such as education, publicity, and advertising, should be used for moral issues as they are for other human resources concerns. Promotional tools are as valuable in reaching the employee group as they are the external market. Their effectiveness can be increased by a professionally designed program. An organization that deliberately promotes morality is likely to get more of it.

8. Leadership should be selected and promoted for both moral and nonmoral competence. An organization can position itself to attract, hire, and promote individuals who pursue moral obligations. The keys to this position include a visible moral concern, systems and procedures noticeably designed to make morality easier, obvious incentives that reward moral performance, and prominent recruiting roles for those who exemplify virtue. But selection requires an abundant supply; the organization must have a surplus of applicants. An organization promoting moral virtue pays competitive wages and builds an attractive work environment to be able to be selective in recruitment and retention.

Obviously, this is not an easy agenda. Yet any community deserves morally excellent health care, and any health care organization can be morally improved. Each of us has the opportunity to make our moral environment either better or worse. Almost any first step will help; the size of the improvement is less important than the initiative. Success feeds on itself. Organizations and individuals whose style supports moral solutions attract people who find the moral challenge an intrinsic reward. Building the momentum meets the moral challenge of health care management at its highest level.

Part IV Epilogue

Follow-up on the Cases

The three institutions involved in these tragedies all survived. Each has striven to become more virtuous, in many instances illustrating the possibilities discussed above.

St. Elizabeth's

St. Elizabeth's has restructured its medical staff peer review, following up on a public promise they made in 1988. Dr. Jon Rahman, chief of the medical staff in 1991, said their peer review procedures are more sophisticated. "'I won't say it's a perfect system. But it is much more intense than ever before.'"[82] They have supported the review process with better data. Computer software analyzes the frequency of procedures and diagnoses and flags physicians with unusual profiles. Rahman said, "'It's meant to be an educational product, not a punitive thing. If somebody's not doing what the other folks are doing and they're getting better results. . . . I think everybody would like to know about it.'"[83]

Commodore Quinn and Captain Hodges*

Navy health care quality management system

The Navy medical department is one of the largest health care systems in existence. More than 50,000 health care professionals, both uniformed and not, provide health care services to a defined population

---

*This section of the epilogue was written by Donald F. Hagen, Vice Admiral, Medical Service Corps, U.S. Navy, Surgeon General of the Navy, and Wynette A. Isley, Lieutenant Commander, Medical Service Corps, U.S. Navy, April 1992. The opinions and assertions in this section are those of the authors and are not to be construed as official or as reflecting the views of the Department of the Navy.

of over 2.7 million people worldwide. The primary mission of the Navy medical department is to provide medical support to the operating naval forces, including the U.S. Marine Corps, during peace and war. In fiscal year 1990, the Navy medical department provided health care in the form of 207,000 admissions, nearly 13 million outpatient visits, and 21,500 births. With a military health care system of such magnitude, the development of sound management systems is essential in the pursuit of quality health care that efficiently and effectively distributes limited resources.

This epilogue describes the Navy prescription for moral behavior, which we define as quality management. Quality health care management implies the right person doing the right thing in the right way at the right place and time. The Navy quality management system measures intended action against documented outcomes. Therefore, a brief overview of the measurement mechanisms that are used to monitor and evaluate the quality of Navy health care is included. The final section describes the organizational culture of the Navy health care system.

The Navy's emerging culture of continuous improvement, called Total Quality Leadership (TQL), supports moral decisions and provides the framework for the Guiding Principles and the vision of the Navy medical department. Like any bureaucratic organization, the Navy health care system is governed by a complex set of written directives, instructions, policies, and procedures. However, the cultural concepts of TQL provide the moral gauge against which to compare an intended action that has not been specifically prescribed. Furthermore, the TQL culture confirms the dignity of each member of the Navy health care team and reinforces the universality of moral law within the Navy health care system.

Quality input: Professional accessions process

The selection of qualified professionals for the Navy health care team is a logical starting point for ensuring quality health care management. The Navy currently has stringent acceptance screening criteria. The accessions process demands quality input into the Navy health care system. Navy recruiters are usually the first contact point for individuals contemplating a professional relationship with the Navy health care system. These recruiters are trained to collect professional credentials documentation, which they forward to recruiting headquarters for preliminary screening. Professional credentials are verified by a civilian company under contract to the Navy. These documents are then forwarded to a central professional review board, which reviews them and interviews the screened applicants. When the health care professional affiliates with the Navy, a summary file of the individual's credentials and privileging status is sent to the first duty station for their official use.

Quality monitoring and evaluation process

Navy health care treatment facilities actively participate in ongoing monitoring and evaluation of care and services, using the JCAHO's Ten Step Process Model[84] and other continuous quality improvement models. Larger Navy treatment facilities (those with more than 25 inpatient beds and those with 100,000 or more annual outpatient visits) are accredited by the JCAHO. In 1990, the average JCAHO accreditation score received by civilian hospitals was 77.2 out of a possible 100. The average score for the Naval hospitals was 86.7 during that same time period. The Navy collects several external indicators to document, in an unbiased and neutral manner, the quality of care provided. The Civilian External Peer Review Program, which is used throughout the Department of Defense, is a retrospective assessment of the quality and appropriateness of care by independent civilian health care professionals under contract to the assistant secretary of defense (Health Affairs). Additionally, the Navy is an active participant in the Maryland Hospital Association Quality Indicator Project, which is a multiyear project to refine the collection and use of appropriate clinical indicators of quality.[85] The results of this project are used as part of the ongoing quality assessment and improvement processes at participating treatment facilities. In each of these assessment processes, Naval hospitals have been evaluated consistently and significantly above the mean.

Quality control: Clinical privileging process

The credentials review and clinical privileging program is an essential element of the Navy quality management system. The Navy recognizes that the quality of health care services depends on the quality of clinical and administrative processes. The potential consequences of actions by unqualified or impaired professionals or by the misconduct of these professionals are so significant that complete verification of credentials and adequate control of clinical privileges is absolutely imperative. The Navy clinical privileging process relies on professional peer review and a prescribed set of documented procedures. Initial privileges are granted based on the credentials verified by the contract agency. Ongoing monitoring and evaluation of health care services provides the feedback loop for quality control. Staff appointments with clinical privileges are reviewed on a two-year cycle with formal clinical performance profiles prepared every six months. Objective, predetermined clinical criteria are compared to observed and documented performance. A series of required reviews by varied officials establishes a system of checks and balances. The system is documented by the comments and signatures of the practitioner, the department head, the chair of the executive committee of the medical staff (after the credentials committee chair, if one is established), and, finally, the signature of the commanding officer as the designated privileging authority or governing body representative.

Total Quality Leadership: The culture of Navy medicine

Total Quality Leadership is the application of quantitative methods and people to assess and improve all significant processes within an organization. In 1988, the Navy surgeon general became personally aware of TQL and was appointed to the Department of the Navy Executive Steering Group. The following year, during their annual meeting, Navy medical department commanding officers learned about this emerging paradigm of quality management. Interest in the application of TQL to the health care field was quickly gaining momentum. In November 1989, Total Quality Management was included in the theme of the annual meeting of the Association of Military Surgeons of the United States. The quality management infrastructure was established at the headquarters of the Navy health care system, the Bureau of Medicine and Surgery, in 1990. That same year saw the development of cultural foundations for the transition to TQL. The newly established Naval Medical Quality Institute developed an implementation roadmap to guide all the Navy medicine on the TQL journey. Forty major medical commands received TQL training in 1991. TQL requires senior management to be educated first, with training then extended down into the organization. This top-down approach is necessary to ensure that decisions made under the TQL paradigm will be morally supported by higher levels in the chain of command.

Conclusion

The tragic occurrence presented earlier in this book can be prevented by a good system of laws and regulations administered by moral leaders.

The Navy health care system is a union of rational beings in a system of common laws. However, it is the organizational culture, not the rules or regulations, that enables or impedes the individual who must act in a moral manner when confronted with an impaired provider. Good leaders establish the organization culture that gives life to the values of that organization. State-of-the-art technology and superior professional education and training, both available in the Navy health care system, must be coupled with a sense of purpose and a clear mission. Leaders, total quality leaders, reinforce the importance of the objectives that support the mission. The Navy health care system has embraced the philosophy of continuous improvement with outstanding leadership, a strong sense of moral purpose, and a clear mission that will stand up to the moral challenges of management.

Blue Cross and Blue Shield of Michigan*

On December 9, 1987, the BCBSM board of directors named Richard E. Whitmer interim CEO and created a search committee to select a new CEO. The following April, the board named Whitmer to the post of permanent president and CEO. At the same time it selected Donald M. D. Thurber, one of the four board members appointed by the governor of the state, as the board chairperson.

Whitmer's selection was in part the result of a position paper that he completed on September 15, 1987, as BCBSM was in the throes of the controversies that led to the end of the McCabe era. Whitmer shared his paper with board members after McCabe stepped down.

Nearly three months before he was to become interim CEO and seven months before he would permanently hold the company's top two jobs, Whitmer wrote that the future prospects of the company could well depend on an honest evaluation of the current state of affairs and an appreciation of the sorts of changes that might be required to maintain future viability. Without prompt attention, the corporation could, at best, drift aimlessly or, at worst, unknowingly blunder off in an altogether wrong and fateful direction, he said.

Whitmer made several key points:

- A successful organization must have a concrete view of itself, and that view must be grounded in reality.

---

*This section of the epilogue was prepared by Blue Cross and Blue Shield of Michigan.

- The CEO is obviously the one person who has more impact on an organization than anyone else.
- All organizations have faults; all have weaknesses. The challenge is not to dwell on them or to assign blame but to correct them.
- What BCBSM needs is a statement of purpose, of mission, that recognizes and reflects the radically restructured business environment in which it operates.
- Blue Cross and Blue Shield of Michigan needs to be well managed, financially sound, cost competitive, and efficient. These characteristics alone, however, might not be enough. The company must also be socially and politically astute.
- Relations with state government must be dramatically changed.
- Relations with Michigan's senior citizens must also be improved.
- The company must create a positive, open, democratic, dynamic, and therefore productive work environment that attracts and keeps quality people.
- The CEO needs immediate credibility.

As soon as he became permanent president and CEO, Whitmer set out to establish credibility for himself and the corporation with a number of key constituencies. He held numerous meetings with the state's insurance commissioner and the attorney general. Ultimately, both addressed the company's board of directors and acknowledged a change in the corporation's direction. Following meetings with editors of major daily newspapers in the state, editorials commended Whitmer's efforts to bring a new attitude to the company and take the corporation in a new direction.

The next major hurdle was the corporation's financial condition, and the perception of regulators that the figures supplied by the company were not valid. Working with regulators, Whitmer arranged for an independent audit by a nationally recognized accounting firm selected by the state. That review confirmed the findings of the company's regular auditors.

Thirty-four changes in corporate accounting and financial procedures recommended by the state's auditors were accepted. Ultimately, all of the company's for-profit subsidiaries were dismantled.

When the corporation's financial statement at the end of the third quarter of 1988 indicated BCBSM was carrying a negative reserve balance, the reports were accepted by everyone with an interest in the company's fiscal position. Fortunately, the company's cash flow was sufficient to carry it for several months. Within three months, by the end of 1988, it had rebuilt its reserves to a modest $29 million. But more was needed. The company announced a $100 million reduction in its administrative expenses over two years including the elimination of 1,400 jobs. This elimination was accomplished through attrition and an early retirement program. Of the 1,400 jobs eliminated, less than 40 were the result of layoffs.

By the end of 1989, reserves reached $278 million. At the end of 1990, they stood at $427 million.

Next a corporate code of business ethics was adopted as well as a corporate mission statement. The code of ethics set standards that precluded even the appearance of any impropriety. The mission statement acknowledged Public Act 350 of 1980 as BCBSM's state governing law and recognized the company's social responsibilities in addition to the need to be competitive and financially sound.

Whitmer next brought a diverse new leadership team to the corporation. The early retirement program gave him the opportunity when a number of senior managers left the company. As a result, a new senior management team was named producing a change of more than 50 percent in corporate leadership with significantly more women and minority members. It was made up of a talented, diverse group who had moved up in the corporate ranks as well as outstanding people brought in from outside the company.

With the new senior management team in place, the company set out to create a new corporate culture for its 7,500 employees to a work style characterized by cooperation, team work, creativity, accountability for results, and determination to provide superior service. A corporate philosophy statement was adopted that articulated Whitmer's belief in teamwork, mutual respect, and good communication both within the corporation and with the outside world. Enhancements to the quality of employee work life were implemented, including day care for children of employees and a program to provide advice and direction for employees who must care for aging parents.

A collective bargaining contract with the UAW, representing 40 percent of the company's work force, was successfully and amicably concluded without a strike in 1990—in contrast to the prolonged work stoppage in 1987.

Totally new participation agreements with hospitals and physicians were developed based on the recommendations of nationally recognized consultants and representatives of the state's hospital and physician community. These included revamped payment mechanisms

148   Improving Virtue

to manage costs and clarifications of long-standing policy issues. All Michigan hospitals signed the new agreement as did seven of every ten physicians in the state.

After ten straight years of declining membership, BCBSM posted a 50,000 gain in membership in 1990. Major initiatives were implemented to improve customer and provider services including new telephone systems with greater capacity and ability to route calls and monitoring of service quality levels. A program to provide free preventive health care for children of the working poor was launched in 1991. It was funded by private donations with BCBSM donating all administrative services.

In three short years, under new leadership the company had taken on a new attitude and headed in a new direction.

Notes to Part IV

1. "Blues Oust Consumer Advocate," *Detroit News*, 23 July 1977.
2. Ibid.
3. "Court Puts Blues Critic Back in Post," *Detroit News*, 20 October 1977.
4. "Consumer Control of Blue Cross Sought," *Detroit News*, 17 December 1977.
5. "Blue Boss Gets $9,000 Pay Raise," *Detroit News*, 9 March 1977.
6. "Blues Spend Millions to Halt Reorganizing," *Detroit News*, 14 September 1980.
7. Ibid.
8. Ibid.
9. Ibid.
10. Ibid.
11. Ibid.
12. Ibid.
13. *Blue Cross & Blue Shield of Michigan v. Governor*, 422 Mich 1 (1985).
14. Ibid.
15. "Blue Cross Seeks Commercial Firm Status," *Detroit News*, 15 September 1983.
16. Ibid.
17. Ibid.
18. Ibid.
19. F. J. Kelley, "State Gives Blues a Fair Shake," *Detroit News*, 25 September 1983, letter to the editor.
20. Ibid.
21. "Blues Hope to Diversify, Spread Risk with Switch," *Detroit News*, 9 October 1983.
22. Ibid.
23. Ibid.
24. Ibid.
25. Ibid.
26. "State Details Blues' 'Illegal' Use of Firms," *Detroit News*, 10 June 1984.
27. Ibid.
28. Ibid.
29. Ibid.
30. Ibid.
31. Ibid.
32. Ibid.
33. Ibid.
34. *Blue Cross & Blue Shield of Michigan*, 422 Mich at 17.
35. Ibid.
36. Ibid. at 27, 19, and 44.
37. "State Eyes Probe of Blues' Funds," *Detroit News*, 27 April 1985.
38. "State Readies Probe of Blues," *Detroit News*, 4 May 1985.
39. Ibid.

150   Improving Virtue

40. Ibid.
41. Ibid.
42. "Blues Claim Harassment by Kelley," *Detroit News*, 1 June 1985.
43. Ibid.
44. "Blues Blame State for $27 Million Loss," *Detroit News*, 28 July 1985.
45. Ibid.
46. "Court Rejects Blues' Appeal," *Detroit News*, 8 October 1985.
47. "Kelley Rips Blues Bosses, Ad Blitz," *Detroit News*, 10 October 1985.
48. "State, Blues Join Battle Once More," *Detroit News*, 28 December 1985.
49. Ibid.
50. Ibid.
51. Ibid.
52. "Blues Investigate McCabe Condo Deals in Florida," *Detroit News*, 29 October 1987.
53. "Audit: McCabe Violated 'Spirit' of Laws," *Detroit News*, 4 December 1987.
54. "Blues Chairman McCabe Asks Board for Early Retirement Deal," *Detroit News*, 9 December 1987.
55. Ibid.
56. "Subsidiaries of Blues Could Be Scrapped," *Detroit News*, 9 January 1988.
57. Ibid.
58. "State Audit Says Blues in Danger of Failing," *Detroit News*, 4 March 1988.
59. Ibid.
60. "Blues Offshotts Cost It Millions," *Detroit News*, 6 March 1988.
61. P. F. Drucker, *Practice of Management* (New York: Harper & Row, 1954).
62. A. F. Southwick, *The Law of Hospital and Health Care Administration*, 2d ed. (Ann Arbor: Health Administration Press, 1988), 585–622.
63. American Hospital Association, *Guide to Hospitals* (Chicago: The Association, 1981–1988).
64. "Ohio Medical Groups Hit for Not Exposing MD's 'Love Surgery,'" *American Medical News*, 27 January 1989.
65. Ibid.
66. "His Peers Waved Red Flags: Monitors' Concern Went Beyond Love Surgery," *Dayton Daily News*, 4 August 1991.
67. *American Medical News*.
68. Ibid.
69. "Charges Against Doctor Bring Ire and Questions," *New York Times* 11 December 1988.
70. *American Medical News*.
71. Southwick, 592.
72. Plato, "The Dialogues of Socrates, Apology," in Plato, *Five Great Dialogues* (New York: Van Nostrand, 1942), 46.
73. Ibid.
74. R. W. Emerson, *Complete Works* (Boston: Houghton, Mifflin, 1903), vol. 2, *Essays*, first series, 212.
75. C. I. Barnard, *The Functions of the Executive* (Cambridge, MA: Harvard University Press, 1954), 82–95.

76. W. K. Frankena, *Ethics*, 2d ed. (Englewood Cliffs, NJ: Prentice-Hall, 1973), 74–75.
77. P. F. Drucker, *The Frontiers of Management: Where Tomorrow's Decisions are Being Shaped* (New York: Truman Talley Books, 1986).
78. W. E. Deming, *Out of Crisis* (Cambridge, MA: Massachusetts Institute of Technology, 1986).
79. J. M. Juran, *Juran on Leadership for Quality: An Executive Handbook* (New York: Free Press, 1989).
80. H. Mintzberg, *The Nature of Managerial Work* (New York: Harper & Row, 1973).
81. Plato.
82. "Checks on Doctors Better, Official Says: St. E's Changed Its Evaluation Process Since TV Expose, Says Chief of Staff," *Dayton Daily News*, 4 August 1991.
83. Ibid.
84. *The Joint Commission Guide to Quality Assurance* (Chicago: The Joint Commission on Accreditation of Healthcare Organizations, 1988), 47–66.
85. S. J. Summer and V. A. Kazandjian, "In Search of Quality: Part IV: The Maryland Hospital Association Quality Indicator Project," *Journal of the American Medical Record Association* 60, no. 10 (1989): 34–38.

About the Author

John R. Griffith, M.B.A., is Andrew Pattullo Collegiate Professor, Department of Health Services Management and Policy, School of Public Health, The University of Michigan. He is a graduate of The Johns Hopkins University and the University of Chicago. Before joining the department in 1960, he was associated with The Johns Hopkins Hospital and Strong Memorial Hospital at the University of Rochester. He was director of the Program and Bureau of Hospital Administration (now part of the Department of Health Services Management and Policy) from 1970 to 1982 and chair of the department from 1987 to 1991.

He has served as president of the Association of University Programs in Health Administration, chairman of the board of Medicus Systems Corporation, and chairman of the board of Health Administration Press. He has been active on the editorial boards for many of the scholarly journals in health care administration. He has been a consultant to federal, state, and local governmental agencies and private hospitals and corporations. Since 1970 he has directed the annual Blue Cross–Blue Shield National Health Care Institute.

Professor Griffith has written numerous articles for both scholarly and professional publications, principally in areas related to improving hospital utilization and productivity, and has authored five books and monographs. *The Well-Managed Community Hospital* was the recipient in 1988 of the James A. Hamilton Hospital Administrators' Book Award, presented by the American College of Healthcare Executives. Professor Griffith received the College's Gold Medal Award in 1992 for his dedication to the advancement of education, for his educational leadership, and for his contributions to health services administration. He is a fellow of the College and a member of the American Public Health Association.